Epistemic Justice in Mental Healthcare

Lisa Bortolotti
Editor

Epistemic Justice
in Mental Healthcare

Recognising Agency and Promoting Virtues Across
the Life Span

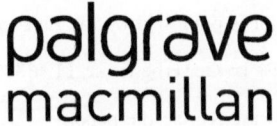

Editor
Lisa Bortolotti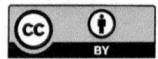
ERI Building
University of Birmingham
Birmingham, UK

ISBN 978-3-031-68880-5   ISBN 978-3-031-68881-2   (eBook)
https://doi.org/10.1007/978-3-031-68881-2

Cover illustration: © Harvey Loake

This Palgrave Macmillan imprint is published by the registered company Springer Nature
Switzerland AG
The registered company address is: Gewerbestrasse 11, 6330 Cham, Switzerland

If disposing of this product, please recycle the paper.

Preface—The Mental Health Patient as a Person, an Agent, and a Partner

This book is a collection of chapters from scientists, clinicians, philosophers, activists, and people with lived experience of mental ill health who identify key challenges for epistemic justice in the context of mental healthcare. The authors propose various strategies to better understand, face, and overcome those challenges. The chapters address issues emerging from mental health crises in the context of serious somatic illness and chronic disease; examine the problems encountered by people with heavily stigmatised symptoms, such as voice hearing and delusions; draw attention to the life-changing impact of mental disorders such as dementia and depression; discuss problematic diagnostic labels such as borderline personality disorders; and review the use of digital health technology. The contributions address practical concerns in healthcare that span the entire life span, from youth to old age, discussing challenging contexts, such as palliative care and care in acute wards. Notwithstanding the variety of themes, there is something that all contributors are equally committed to do, and that is to encourage us to think carefully and critically about our mutual relationships in clinical encounters, promoting a reflection on what it means to be a mental health patient. That is the purpose of project EPIC (Epistemic Injustice in Healthcare, 2023–2029), generously funded by a Wellcome Discovery Award and led by Havi Carel at the University of Bristol. It is thanks to project EPIC that this book can be made available open access.

Every time we meet and talk to each other, we exchange information. In successful social interactions we have an opportunity to exercise our agency by pursuing goals which might include acquiring relevant information and sharing it with others, making informed decisions, solving problems, and generally gaining a better understanding of ourselves and the world around us. We call those goals *epistemic*, because they have to do with exchanging and obtaining knowledge.

Epistemic justice is threatened when certain aspects of our identities (e.g. our age, gender, race, socio-economic status, health, etc.) trigger negative stereotypes that cause others to dismiss our perspective and underestimate our capacity to produce and share knowledge. Often the assumption is that, if we need support with our mental health, the capacities that support our *epistemic agency* are compromised. In the case of serious mental illness, the default assumption is that we lack epistemic agency altogether; in other words, we no longer have the capacity to produce and share knowledge about ourselves and the world, and thus we cannot contribute to shared problem-solving and decision-making. This assumption does not go unchallenged because mental illness and irrationality have been perceived as intertwined. The idea that, if we are mentally ill, then we must be irrational, and thus we cannot be good epistemic agents, is still prevalent in popular culture.

When we take up the role of the patient who accesses services, we are already in a vulnerable position. We are in need of support and, in most cases, we need to rely on other people's technical expertise and clinical experience in order to find the best way to address the problems that we face. These problems can often be understood as a threat to our sense of agency. "Patient" come from *pathos*, which is translated as "suffering". *Pathos* is about being subject to something (usually bad), undergoing, or experiencing (pain or death). There is nothing active or agentive in suffering, it is an experience that happens to us and that, typically, we do not choose to have. Moreover, it is something that often prevents us from doing what we want to do. When there is inflammation in our lower back, we may no longer be able to lift our suitcase or carry our child. When we have a serious injury or need complex medical tests or treatment, we may be confined to a hospital room, and the demands of the life we are used to may have to wait. These experiences result in our feeling like a burden to others, helpless, dependent, weak.

But in addition to what ill health does to us, our role as patients may give rise to further disempowerment. Unless we are also medical practitioners in the relevant area, when we are patients, we are in a subordinate epistemic position with respect to the healthcare professional in the power dynamic of the clinical interaction. As patients we need resources; the healthcare professional is the gateway to such resources. As patients we typically lack competence required to offer adequate causal explanations for what is happening to us, and we are not in a position to propose solutions; the healthcare professional is medically trained and has the clinical experience required to offer those explanations and propose those solutions.

This book discusses and addresses the further threats to our agency that we may have to face when we access mental healthcare. Our role as patients should not rule out the possibility that we play other roles, as *persons* with values, needs, and interests that matter; as *agents* with a perspective on life that deserves validation, and the capacity to share knowledge; and as *partners* in the projects of identifying problems, finding solutions, and making decisions about our future health journey. The knowledge we can share about ourselves, our lives, our health, and our participation in the problem-solving and decision-making that happens during the clinical encounter is central to the success of that encounter.

The medical goal of the clinical encounter, that is, identifying solutions to the patient's health problems, cannot be achieved satisfactorily without (1) fostering mutual trust between patient and practitioner; (2) foregrounding the patient's needs and interests so that the best course of action can be taken moving forward; and (3) counteracting the patient's sense of disempowerment. These desiderata are especially hard to achieve in mental healthcare, where the default assumption too often still is that the need to address our distress as patients trumps our values, needs, and interests; that our perspectives (experiences, beliefs, emotions) may be products of our distress; and that we cannot contribute to identifying problems, finding solutions, and making decisions about our future health journey because our distress compromises our overall rationality, autonomy, and overall capacity. In this book, contributors highlight how harmful it is to forget that, even as mental health patients, we remain persons whose sense of agency may be threatened by illness and distress but needs to be sustained in clinical encounters to enable us to achieve better health outcomes.

As patients, we can also play the role of partners and collaborators in epistemic enterprises led by healthcare professionals, aimed at understanding what might be happening to us and finding the best means of support. And not only can we play those roles, but our contributions are important, because we are the experts in how it feels to have the health problem that we do have, and in how that particular health problem is affecting our lives. Osteoarthritis has a more devastating effect on a pianist's career than a physicist's, and infertility is a bigger issue for a person who wants to have their own biological children than for a person who does not. Health problems need to be understood in the context of a person's values, needs, and interests. Enabling patients to become involved in planning and shared decision-making is not just an opportunity for the healthcare practitioner to treat the patient with respect and make them feel that their perspective is valued, but it is important for the success of the clinical interaction, in terms of contributing to the quality of the therapeutic relationship and increasing the chance that positive health outcomes can be achieved.

In this volume, contributors are experts occupying multiple roles at once (mental health patient, practitioner, academic, researcher, lived experience expert, and activist) and teaming up with other experts from complementary disciplinary areas and areas of expertise in order to offer analyses that take into account various dimensions of epistemic justice, such as being understood, being trusted, having the opportunity to contribute to positive change, being included in shared decision-making, finding meaning in life, and living and dying with dignity. The book's emphasis is on the importance of healthcare practitioners and patients working together to identify the harms of epistemic unjust behaviours and harness existing knowledge and experience to remedy such harms.

The hope is that further research in the areas explored in the book will lead to concrete changes that benefit patients across the life span by supporting healthcare professionals in employing effective communication techniques, welcoming patient advocacy, and gaining expertise and fluency in methods of coauthorship and coproduction.

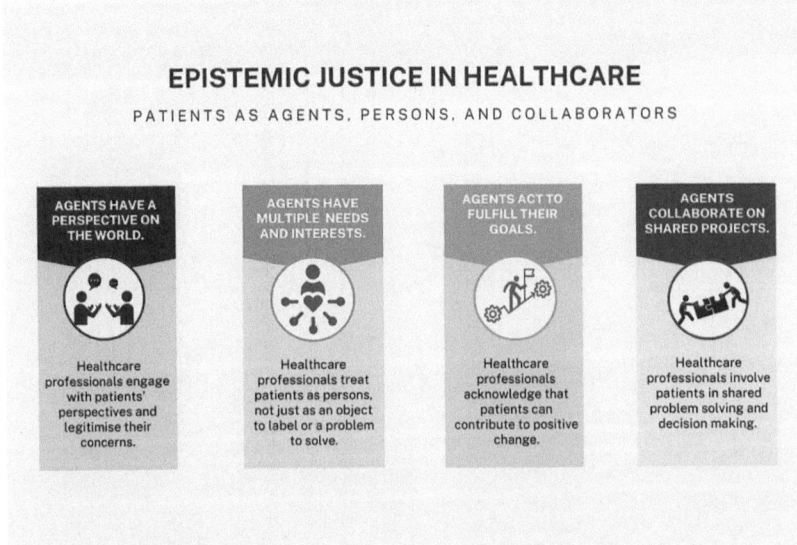

Fig. 1   Epistemic Justice in Healthcare

Birmingham, UK

Lisa Bortolotti
Matthew Broome

Contents

List of Contributors

Martino Belvederi Murri Institute of Psychiatry, Department of Neuroscience and Rehabilitation, University of Ferrara, Ferrara, Italy

Lisa Bortolotti Department of Philosophy and Institute for Mental Health, University of Birmingham, Birmingham, UK

Owen Braid The Voice Collective, Mind in Camden, London, UK

Matthew Broome Institute for Mental Health, University of Birmingham, Birmingham, UK

Rosangela Caruso Institute of Psychiatry, Department of Neuroscience and Rehabilitation, University of Ferrara, Ferrara, Italy

Rabih Chattat Department of Psychology, University of Bologna, Bologna, Italy

Ilaria Chirico Department of Psychology, University of Bologna, Bologna, Italy

Josh Cottrell McPin Foundation, London, UK

Shioma-Lei Craythorne Aston Institute of Health & Neurodevelopment, Aston University, Birmingham, UK

Marco Cruciata Institute of Psychiatry, Department of Neuroscience and Rehabilitation, University of Ferrara, Ferrara, Italy

Catherine Fadashe McPin Foundation, London, UK

Federica Folesani Department of Neuroscience and Rehabilitation, University of Ferrara, Ferrara, Italy

Luigi Grassi Institute of Psychiatry, Department of Neuroscience and Rehabilitation, University of Ferrara, Ferrara, Italy

Gurpriya Kapoor The Voice Collective, Mind in Camden, London, UK

Elisabetta Lalumera Department for Life Quality Studies, University of Bologna, Rimini, Italy

Michael Larkin Aston Institute of Health & Neurodevelopment, Aston University, Birmingham, UK

Michele Lim McPin Foundation, London, UK

Fiona Malpass The Voice Collective, Mind in Camden, London, UK

Rose McCabe School of Health and Psychological Sciences, City, University of London, London, UK

Kathleen Murphy-Hollies Philosophy Department, University of Birmingham, Birmingham, UK

Maria Giulia Nanni Department of Neuroscience and Rehabilitation, University of Ferrara, Ferrara, Italy

Eleanor Palafox-Harris Department of Philosophy, University of Birmingham, Birmingham, UK

Oscar Sharples McPin Foundation, London, UK

Chris Sims McPin Foundation, London, UK

Thalia Somerville-Large The Voice Collective, Mind in Camden, London, UK

Rachel Temple McPin Foundation, London, UK

Sara Trolese Department of Psychology, University of Bologna, Bologna, Italy

Jay Watts Centre for Mental Health Research, City, University of London, London, UK

LIST OF TABLES

Being Understood: Epistemic Injustice Towards Young People Seeking Support for Their Mental Health

Michael Larkin, *Rose McCabe*, *Lisa Bortolotti*,
Matthew Broome, *Shioma-Lei Craythorne*,
Rachel Temple, *Michele Lim*, *Catherine Fadashe*,
*Chris Sims, Oscar Sharples, Josh Cottrell, as part of the Agency
in Practice team*

Abstract Across many domains, it is important for us to feel that we are understood by others. This is crucial when we are disclosing a vulnerability or seeking help for a problem. When these disclosures or help-seeking requests relate to *mental health difficulties*, our interactions with others can carry many threats, including stigmatisation; inappropriate moral or character judgements; overly stringent threshold evaluations; and

The Agency-in-Practice team is comprised of psychologists, linguists, philosophers, psychiatrists, and young people with experiences of accessing mental health services and conducting research. From 2022 to 2024 they were

M. Larkin (✉) · S.-L. Craythorne
Aston Institute of Health & Neurodevelopment, Aston University, Birmingham,

© The Author(s) 2025
L. Bortolotti (ed.), *Epistemic Justice in Mental Healthcare*,
https://doi.org/10.1007/978-3-031-68881-2_1

assumptions about our personal circumstances and social resources. In this chapter, we summarise some of the core findings from empirical and qualitative studies which examine what happens when young people meet with health professionals to disclose or to seek help for their experiences with poor mental health. We then draw out some key implications for improving relational and communicative practices amongst mental health professionals. We focus on those implications which are highlighted by those members of our team who are young adults with experiences of accessing mental health services and reflect on these implications in the light of insights from the literature on epistemic injustice.

Keywords Youth · Mental health · Felt understanding · Agency · Clinical encounters

UK
e-mail: m.larkin@aston.ac.uk

R. McCabe
School of Health and Psychological Sciences, City, University of London, London, UK

L. Bortolotti
Philosophy Department and Institute for Mental Health, University of Birmingham, Birmingham, UK

R. Temple · M. Lim · C. Fadashe · C. Sims · O. Sharples · J. Cottrell
McPin Foundation, London, UK

M. Broome
Institute for Mental Health, University of Birmingham, Birmingham, UK

funded by a UKRI Methodology grant to develop a participatory methodology for analysing qualitative mental health data with young people as co-analysts. The team includes corresponding author Michael Larkin (School of Psychology, Aston University. Email: m.larkin@aston.ac.uk. ORCID: 0000-0003-3304-7000), Rose McCabe, Lisa Bortolotti, Matthew Broome, Shioma-Lei Craythorne, Rachel Temple, Michele Lim, Catherine Fadashe, Chris Sims, Oscar Sharples, Josh Cottrell and additional members of the Young Person's Advisory Group at the McPin Foundation.

1.1 What Is Known About Young People's Experiences of Disclosure and Help-Seeking?

Social relations are at risk when communicative systems break down, and mutual understanding is lost. In the context of mental healthcare, the success of interventions and services relies upon co-operative relationships. To benefit from such support structures, the users of services must feel that they can trust the intentions and actions of the staff who provide them with care. In turn, staff need to gather clinically relevant information from patients, so that they can understand the problem, predict what might happen, and plan interventions accordingly.

For many young people, the sense of being understood is a precursor to being able to develop the trust that is, in turn, necessary for any sort of engagement with assessment and intervention. When people feel that their needs and feelings have *not* been properly understood by professionals, those professionals' attempts to build trust and provide meaningful support are likely to fail. A person's (or family's) capacity for withstanding crises is thus linked to social processes of understanding, and specifically, the feeling of *being understood*. This feeling is consistently associated with feelings of social connectedness and wellbeing; conversely, the feeling of *not* being understood is a corollary of negative emotions and poorer life satisfaction (Oishi et al., 2008, 2010).

Experimental studies have emphasised that 'felt understanding' is a social phenomenon, with both cognitive and emotional components (Morelli et al., 2014), and that many environmental factors (above and beyond whether we have actually *been* 'understood') contribute to whether we are likely to experience a sense of 'felt understanding' (Reis et al., 2017). Situational obstructions to 'felt understanding' are particularly important in those mental health interactions when we meet with professionals to disclose difficulties and seek help. Such obstructions are features of the context and relationship which impede mutual understanding. For example, in these situations, there is a lot at stake, there are vulnerabilities to be exposed, and the two parties may each have different priorities and access to different kinds of knowledge about the problem.

The sense that we are being understood is thus especially crucial when we are disclosing that we are struggling with something, because people who understand us may be more likely to respond sympathetically. Similarly, when we are seeking help for a problem, we want to speak to people who understand us because they may be more likely to offer meaningful help. When these disclosures or help-seeking requests relate to *mental health difficulties*, our interactions with others can come with risks. These risks include stigmatisation; inappropriate moral or character judgements; overly stringent threshold evaluations ('you're not *really* ill'); and assumptions about our personal circumstances and social resources ('ask someone at home to help you'). These ultimately may lead to worse mental health outcomes for the individual seeking help.

Lack of trust and the feeling of not being understood are both likely to lead to disengagement from services or delays in help-seeking. The former are likely to be associated with worse experiences of services, and the latter with worse outcomes.

1.2   WHAT ARE THE KEY IMPLICATIONS FOR IMPROVING RELATIONAL AND COMMUNICATIVE PRACTICES AMONGST MENTAL HEALTH PROFESSIONALS?

In our research, we have been working together as an interdisciplinary team of young people with lived experience and academic researchers from psychology, philosophy, linguistics, clinical communication, and psychiatry. We have found two concepts—epistemic injustice and agency—to be particularly helpful in thinking about what can go well, and what can go wrong, during encounters between clinicians and young people seeking help for their mental health (Bergen et al., 2022, 2023). As an orienting concept, epistemic injustice has resonated strongly with the young people in our team, allowing us to identify many aspects of what can go wrong during real-world help-seeking encounters.

In our meetings together, we have observed and discussed audio and video recordings of situations in which young people sought help from professionals. We saw that often they were not listened to, were not asked the right questions, were assumed to be capable (or incapable) of various kinds of coping without the professionals establishing whether this was the case, and were assumed to have (or not have) various kinds of knowledge which was not properly discussed. These present major barriers to 'being understood', the development of trust, and the subsequent delivery of care in any healthcare setting. In mental healthcare, where the *relationship* with the healthcare professional *is a part of* the therapeutic care provided, the barrier is especially problematic.

As a means of addressing these problems, and beginning to think about our aspirations for what could go well (or sometimes, *did* go well), agency has been a useful corollary to epistemic injustice: young people in our team have been keen to think about 'best practice' in terms of how professionals might support young people to have access to more information and knowledge, to have more choice (and the opportunity to act upon it), and to be more involved in their care and treatment-planning.

To support this, it is possible to make practical recommendations from existing evidence about what clinicians can do in their communication with young people, to ensure that these encounters are more likely to go well. These observations and recommendations are based on analysing audio and video recordings of mental health encounters between young people and mental health professionals. The interactions took place in hospital Accident and Emergency departments and were conducted by mental health liaison teams. To understand the interactions, we drew on an analytic method called conversation analysis. Conversation analysis involves micro-analysing verbal and non-verbal communication, focusing on what people say and how they say it. Some recommendations are also based on interviews with people and professionals about what went well and what did not go so well in these encounters.

Many (if not all) mental health encounters involve delicate and emotional conversations. People receiving mental healthcare report that the therapeutic relationship and trust are central to these conversations as they often feel shame and stigma (Radez et al., 2021). A good therapeutic relationship is characterised by feeling that the professional understands the meaning of your experiences, cares about you and is not just 'doing their job'. While many of the critical elements that underpin a good therapeutic relationship—such as curiosity, listening, and validation of the person's experiences—sound straightforward, achieving them in practice is not (Bortolotti & Murphy-Hollies, 2023).

Questions are fundamental to understanding the quality of mental health encounters. Mental health professionals ask a lot of questions. In any interaction, the person who asks the questions sets the agenda for the interaction (e.g. professional-patient, teacher-student, manager-employee). Initially, asking questions sounds like it is consistent with being curious. However, being curious involves an open stance that is reflected in the kinds of questions asked and how they are asked. Conversation analysis of actual recordings shows how the design of questions impacts the ways in which young people can respond (e.g. McCabe et al.,

2023): questions can be demonstrably open, or they can have constraints built into them. For example, consider these two opening questions to a psychosocial assessment after a mental health crisis presentation to the Emergency Department (ED):

- "So what- obviously I've seen in the notes- We've seen a bit in- in the medical notes about what's happened. Got a bit of a background. But it's really important for us to hear in your words....[open arm gesture]"

versus

- "I've had a look at the hospital notes here today em.... So what I'll do is I'll talk to you about why you're here today. So I understand that you've taken quite a large overdose? Of ibuprofen? Can you tell me a little bit about what led up to that?"

These two questions have very different impacts on what the person discloses in each case. In the first case, the person went on to provide an extensive narrative about the events leading up to their ED attendance. In the second case, the person responded with much less information about what led up to the overdose.

The kinds of questions that professionals ask indicate how open the agenda will be. In the first example above, the agenda is open, and the professional is inviting the person to tell their story ("Got a bit of a background. But it's really important for us to hear in your words") whereas in the second example, the person is invited to tell a more limited version of their story ("Can you tell me a little bit about what led up to that [the overdose]?"). There is a tension here between giving people the opportunity to tell their story and protecting them from the frustration of having to re-tell it on multiple occasions. There might be some situations in which some of the young person's story is already known to the professional, and then of course, it would be appropriate to pitch the question accordingly. The key point is that questions set the agenda in very specific ways: each question makes a certain type of response (and not others) relevant. Questions that encourage the person to talk about what is important to them include:

- Can you tell me more about that?
- When did all this start for you?
- What else has been happening in your life?
- Reflecting back what the person has said 'So you're feeling worried about that?' to encourage expansion, and/or check that one has understood.

When asked in a sensitive and open manner, these questions can provide an opportunity for a young person to describe and expand upon their experience. Questioning is part of listening because it constrains (or not) what can be said and hence what can be heard. More open questions display curiosity and tend to occur with more active listening. In routine mental healthcare, listening can be difficult as the focus is typically on 'assessing' a person's mental state. In an assessment interview structure, the format tends to be question–answer, with no conversational slots for listener feedback. For this reason, the structure involves the clinician continuing to ask questions rather than actively listening to what people are saying. Active listening includes:

Open posture and leaning forward (rather than leaning back, e.g. with arms folded)

- Eye contact
- Allowing time for people to respond and possibly expand on their responses
- Not interrupting
- Giving non-verbal feedback such as nodding while the person is speaking, or having an engaged tone of voice that is congruent with the subject matter (i.e. sounding empathetic when a young person is discussing a particularly vulnerable topic)

1.3   WHAT IS MOST IMPORTANT TO YOUNG ADULTS WITH EXPERIENCES OF ACCESSING MENTAL HEALTH SERVICES?

As will be evident, the gap between 'what goes well' and 'what goes wrong' cannot be entirely bridged by improvements in communication skills. Our concerns about addressing epistemic injustice and improving young people's agency during help-seeking also require us to think about issues related to trust, power, fairness, control, and choice, for example. Having outlined what is known about the problem above, we asked the young people in our team to identify their key questions for clinical and conceptual development in this area. In the remaining two sections of the chapter, we discuss these priority concerns.

1.3.1   What Are the Things That You Can Do to Ensure a Young Person Feels Understood?

As we have seen in the previous section, taking care to ask the right questions, and making sure that these questions are asked in the right way, is crucial. For young people to feel understood, they need first to be provided with an opportunity to tell their story, and to do so in a way which feels safe, which can contain and tolerate their distress, and which is open to the complexity of the situation as they see it. This obviously extends beyond what the professional asks and reaches further, to cover the way that they react to the young person's account.

Validating peoples' experiences when they are feeling very vulnerable is important, because they may feel very unsure and uncertain about what is happening to them. When we watched video recordings of mental health encounters, the young people in our team found it striking how little validation there was for people's distress. Validation of difficult experiences and distress can be achieved without extending the length of the encounter (Bergen et al., 2022). Examples of validation are:

- 'It sounds like you've been going through a really challenging time'.
- 'That's a really difficult place to be in'.
- 'That's a [e.g. scary/sad/difficult/overwhelming] thought'.

Young people can worry about being perceived as 'time-wasters', so validating their help-seeking can be reassuring—e.g. 'Thank you for sharing all of this with me. You did the right thing by coming here today. We are here to support you through this'. Likewise, this can create a sense of safety through being acknowledged, that allows the young person to further open up about their experiences—facilitating further sharing of information between them and the healthcare professional.

What was often the case when the team reviewed the clinical encounter was that we observed a dialogue that appeared more quasi-legal than therapeutic, with clinicians citing evidence which undercut or discounted the testimony of the young people. For example, a young person seeking help with feelings of suicidality was told that they could not in fact be feeling suicidal, because they had revealed that they had plans to attend a social event.

Two reflections we made as a team included that, first, mental health nurses often may see multiple young people, in acute distress, back-to-back and without a break or opportunity for supervisory support. This could lead to feelings of emotional disconnectedness and compassion fatigue. Second, the practitioners were working in a system where there was a marked constraint in the services and resources that could be offered. We wondered if this tended to distort the assessments themselves (it is uncomfortable to be in a situation where help is needed and cannot be provided—e.g. see Williamson et al., 2021 on moral injury) by setting a starting assumption that enhanced support would generally not be required (e.g. see Strech et al., 2008 on the phenomena of 'bedside rationing').

1.3.2   Who Should Be Involved in Deciding on Diagnosis and How Should the Process Be Carried Out?

A direct response to this question is simply to say: the patient and the professional. Shared decision-making has been an established principle of healthcare for some time, but its journey from principle to practice has not been seamless. The idea is simply that patients have a right to be involved in decisions about their care, and that patients and professionals should work together to decide on the right treatment. Most people reading this will probably be able to think of at least one time when they felt that this is what happened, and at least one time when it definitely did not!

One of the reasons that is sometimes given for the slow progress in making shared decision-making a part of routine practice is that the evidence is unclear about whether it makes a difference to treatment outcomes. This is because there is insufficient high-quality research evidence to allow us to draw firm conclusions about that aspect (see Aoki et al., 2022). However, as Slade (2017) and others have pointed out, one of the most important reasons for taking this approach is an ethical one (i.e. it is the right and just thing to do, as we discuss below). Interestingly, the evidence does suggest that clinical work based around shared decision-making approaches does *not* take significantly longer (Cruz & Pincus, 2002; Légaré et al., 2010, 2012). This certainly resonates with our observations that relatively simple changes to professionals' questioning style can have a big impact on whether a person feels understood (e.g. see Shay & Lafata, 2015) and is then able to actively engage in a discussion and decision about their care. There is emerging evidence from adolescents and families that shared decision-making can help with finding treatments that are acceptable (e.g. see Bjønness et al., 2020), and which young people are therefore more likely to engage with.

This does highlight an additional issue. For many young people, there are other people (parents, carers) who may feel they should have a say in the decision-making process. Sometimes this can be helpful and may be experienced as such by the young person. Sometimes it may be unhelpful or experienced as intrusive. While there are some age-related legal limitations around this, professionals often have to make a clinical decision with the young person about when and how to involve family members. For clinicians, they can maintain confidentiality to a young person, but still allow a parent or carer to offer their views, if the young person is willing. A helpful strategy can be to see the young person alone, then with the family member, and to clarify with young person what information they are happy to have shared with the parent/carer. Parents can also be nervous when their child is seen by mental health professional—they may be concerned about being blamed for the young person's distress and can be anxious about social services and children being taken into care. These anxieties can limit the open-ness of discussion.

1.3.3   *What Do Young People Need to Know About the Treatment That Is on Offer?*

This interesting question leads us in a couple of different directions. On the one hand, there is an extensive research literature on 'mental health literacy'. This literature focuses on developing measures of people's knowledge and understanding of mental health issues, and on developing and delivering interventions to improve their knowledge and understanding (e.g. see Nobre et al., 2021; Patafio et al., 2021; Seedaket et al., 2020). Often the focus is on knowing enough about the kinds of problems which mental health professionals can help with, in order to seek help in a timely and appropriate fashion. To some extent this is a developmental question, because we might expect an 18-year-old to need to know more than an 8-year-old (e.g. see Kågström et al., 2023), but it is also a contextual matter, because different populations have access to different care (McGorry et al., 2022).

Knowing that it is possible or wise to seek help from mental health professionals is generally contrasted with knowledge that might lead young people to seek help elsewhere, such as from spiritual leaders or traditional healers (e.g. see Renwick et al., 2022), so the concept of literacy here includes a judgement about which kinds of knowledge are 'best'. In this respect, the analogy with 'literacy' is a little misleading: this field of research is concerned with differentiating between the 'right' and 'wrong' ways of understanding mental health, as seen through the lens of an evidence-based medicine approach. In mental health, there will be differences of opinion even within and between different forms of evidence-based practice. This can be difficult to get to grips with, especially if one is not feeling well, and/or not familiar with the key concepts and terms. Providing information and understanding of the issues which might usefully guide one's help-seeking choices (e.g. through psychoeducation materials) can be a helpful way to support young people as they navigate their way through this.

When we examine clinical encounters, we notice that a conventional focus on *help-seeking* means that the literature is pointing towards something which has already happened. It is generally unclear on what a 'good enough' standard of mental health literacy might be, in order for someone to actively engage in negotiating what their own *care and treatment* should look like. For those kinds of insights, we need to turn to the literature from survivors and experts-by-experience, who have produced materials to help others to know what to ask about, what to ask for (e.g. see Faulkner, 2020), what to share, and even what to pack in one's bag (e.g. see Anderson, 2022). There are also 'how to' guides produced by therapists and professionals, who have written about the different kinds of therapy which are available. There are far fewer of these kinds of resources for young people than there are for adults (but see Selby, 2019, for a notable exception). In our project, some of our young colleagues have been making videos to help share information about what to expect and what to ask.[1]

The second interesting angle relates to what a young person might actually need to understand, in order to engage effectively in the kinds of shared decision-making described in the previous sub-section. In clinical interactions, we might generally think of these needs less in terms of a level of 'literacy' in mental-health-as-topic, and more in terms of a degree of 'capacity' to understand what is at stake. Traditionally—and legally—professionals have focused primarily on the capacity of the person to understand what is being discussed and to express choices and make decisions. But as we have seen above, there is also the matter of the capacity of the professional to: (a) facilitate the young person's involvement in the discussion and (b) make themselves understood.

This is important because the burden of 'knowing enough' ought not to fall upon the young person, before they are able to engage in thinking with clinicians about their treatment and support. The clinician's role involves taking care to establish what the young person already knows and understands, and then ensuring that they explain anything else that is relevant in accessible and appropriate terms. This should always be a part of the conversation about the problem, and about the next steps in responding to that problem. This is a less straightforward issue than it may first appear, because of the effects of power imbalances, and because agency is a dynamic and complex phenomenon, as we explore further in the following sections.

Finally, it is important to be realistic and accurate in the information which we share. Young people will—quite rightly—withdraw their trust if they are promised help which they cannot access, which does not meet their needs, or which is not available.

1.4   Reflections in the Light of Insights from the Literature on Epistemic Injustice

In our work, the notion of epistemic injustice is mostly explored in the context of clinical encounters, where it is entwined with a range of other aspects of inequality and power. In all interactions where one party has

---

[1] To watch the videos, follow this link: https://collaborativeresearch.co.uk/agency-in-practice.

more authority and power than the other party, there is a risk that the contribution of the party considered less authoritative and powerful is not sought at all or is undervalued and dismissed. Examples include the relationships between parent and child, and teacher and student. Sources of perceived authority can vary: in the teacher/student relationship, teachers are the most authoritative party in virtue of their training, role, and expertise. In the parent/child relationship, parents are typically the most authoritative party in virtue of their age, role, and responsibility—although roles can be reversed in situations where decisions that impact on the parents' lives are made by their adult children when the parents are incapacitated.

Power in part reflects that fact that one party is the gateway to the other party's access to desirable goods and resources. Teachers can write reports and references that may contribute to determine the students' further academic trajectory. Parents can facilitate or obstruct their children's pursuit of certain goals in personal relationships, career, and other interests. In the case of interactions between young people who experience poor mental health and mental healthcare professionals, the source of the authority is the professionals' expertise and special role in providing a diagnosis, recommending a treatment, and offering access to further sources of support. Other factors can come into play, as with all other asymmetrical relationships, and two of them seem to be extremely relevant in this context: *age* and *perceived agency*.

Amongst the young people in our team there is curiosity about what can be done to avoid epistemic injustice more broadly, especially as the issues that might affect a young person's sense of agency are not confined to their struggle with mental health and their exchanges with healthcare professionals.

Any figures of authority and potential sources of support in a young person's life, such as parents, guardians, family members, teachers, employers, may be called upon to safeguard the young person's sense of agency. They can do this by validating their experiences, recognising their concerns, avoiding blame, and involving them in decision-making.

Often, this may require finding a common ground between the young person's understanding of their own experience and a third-party perspective that might be significantly different. Although the lens through which we look at the young person's problem may be instrumental to the choice of strategy we adopt to offer support or attempt to resolve the crisis, all strategies can include a consideration of how the young person can be empowered in their personal journey and build a narrative that is meaningful to them and helps them make sense of their experiences. This kind of empowered agency, or 'critical consciousness', is associated with improved wellbeing (Maker Castro et al., 2022).

1.4.1   How Can We Make Sure That Encounters Between Young People and Professionals Are Fair?

When a young person accesses services for their mental health, they are often experiencing a crisis. Why is this relevant? They already are in a subordinate position due to their young age, which is usually associated with negative stereotypes such as being inexperienced and unreliable, seeking attention, and lacking stability (Houlders et al., 2021). But they are also seen as potentially lacking agency. Common assumptions are that people who experience poor mental health (1) have a perspective on the world that may be distorted; (2) have concerns that may not be justified; (3) are first and foremost a problem to be fixed; (4) cannot contribute to positive change in their lives; (5) are unable to fully participate in decision-making processes (Bergen et al., 2022). This is due to a pre-theoretical tendency to identify mental health with rationality and autonomy, and mental ill health with irrationality and lack of capacity (Bortolotti, 2013). This tendency is misleading. When we experience poor mental health, we may see reality differently from other people, we experience distress and difficulties in communicating and functioning, and we may need more support to pursue our goals. This does not mean, by default, that our perspectives lack value (or cannot offer important insights), that our reports are unreliable, or that we cannot pursue our goals effectively with support.

So, a first step to promote fairer and more productive exchanges in the clinical encounter is to pre-empt the risks of the application of negative stereotypes, which can bring what we may call *epistemic injustice* (Kidd et al., 2022). The sort of epistemic injustice we are thinking about in this context occurs when the testimony of a person in an exchange is dismissed due to a negative stereotype associated with the person's identity (such as being a young person struggling with their mood). Epistemic injustice is at play when the most authoritative and powerful party (the mental healthcare professional) sees the other party (a young person experiencing a mental health crisis) as lacking agency. The problem is that the practitioner may see the young person as a cluster of symptoms in search for a diagnostic label, dismissing their potential contributions to the exchange (Bergen et al., 2023).

The tendency to perceive someone as lacking agency is a more common sort of behaviour than we might think, and if mental health-care professionals sometimes have this tendency, they are definitely not alone. We are all tempted to believe that someone who endorses views that are significantly different from ours is 'out of their mind' or 'makes no sense'. These common expressions suggest that we are not seeing the other person as merely being 'mistaken about something', but as being an unworthy companion in our pursuit of the truth. We stop trusting them and suspend or question our assumption that they can exercise agency. A similar dynamic can emerge between young people and healthcare professionals in instances where a young person's experience of a mental health difficulty may diverge from a practitioner's own expectations or notions.

It might be beneficial in these contexts to remind both parties in an asymmetrical exchange that the best policy is always the adoption of the agential stance. The agential stance is a set of assumptions. When we commit to it, we commit to seeing the other person as (1) having a valuable perspective on the world (even if we end up not sharing that perspective); (2) having legitimate concerns that we should address (even if it is initially difficult for us to understand those concerns); (3) being a person with a complex set of interests and needs, and not merely a problem to be fixed; (4) having the capacity to contribute to positive change, with adequate support; and (5) being able to participate in a process of decision-making about their future, with adequate support (Bergen et al., 2022). We think that this is a good formulation because it can be helpful even when the person's view of their own agency is troubled and dynamic (e.g. see Stone et al., 2020).

In practice, what does the adoption of the agential stance imply? It is an invitation for practitioners to listen attentively and with empathy to what young people have to say, without assuming that what is being said is necessarily a product of illness, and to ask probing questions to better appreciate where the young people's perspective comes from. Reminding people of the importance of adopting the agential stance should also be seen as a warning: if the young person does not have the opportunity to express their views and voice their concerns, they cannot share knowledge that may be instrumental to understanding their situation better and to offering them the best available advice and treatment.

1.4.2   How Can We Make Sure That Young People Retain Control over Their Lives in Their Relationship with Mental Health Services?

Most of the literature on the relationship between patients and practitioners focuses on what practitioners should do to make sure that patients are heard (see e.g. Crichton et al., 2017), and in our answer to the previous question we were guilty of focusing on that too. We suggested that mental healthcare professionals should adopt the agential stance in interactions with young people struggling with their mental health.

But what can young people do to support their own sense of agency and thereby also feel that they retain some control over their lives even at critical times? Can they protect their sense of agency while they are struggling with their mental health? First, it is helpful to change our general attitude towards agency. We tend to assume that agency is a gift we may have or lose, something that can be ON and give us control or can be OFF and leave us helpless. The notion of agency has been idealised in misleading ways, resulting in the feeling that being an agent is like being a lone ranger or a superhero, loaded with awesome powers but overburdened with responsibilities.

Especially in the context of discussion about responsibility, philosophers have often depicted as an individual's affirmation of mastery over the world and of independence with respect to other agents' wills. Either *I really wanted to buy that roasted chicken* or *I was brainwashed to do it*. But real-life agents are neither superheroes nor puppets. They are something in-between. Maybe I craved some meat for dinner tonight and it was passing in front of a fried chicken shop on the way home that made me think of chicken instead of beef? Our behaviour can be driven by our goals but is also shaped by a number of other factors, sometimes known to us and at other times quite hard to detect. There are some powers involved of course, such as the capacity to contribute to change and to participate in decision-making, that we can exercise in favourable circumstances, but even these modest powers are clearly constrained by what opportunities are afforded to us by the surrounding physical and social environment.

Challenges to individualistic and idealised agency come from various sources. According to feminist critiques of traditional accounts of agency, interpersonal relationships are often neglected in how agents are traditionally characterised. For Westlund (2009) we cannot have autonomous agency unless we are open to the reflection that comes from dialogue with others. Another threat to agency comes from the empirical studies on what predicts people's behaviour (Doris, 2002), suggesting that our professed intentions and character traits do not determine how we act and what we decide. The claim is that contextual features of the situation in which we find ourselves have a great influence on our behaviour. This aligns with concepts mapped out in the literature on relational agency (Burkitt, 2018). Burkitt's view is that the capacity for action is a product of one's relationship to others (as enabled and/or constrained by power differentials). He specifically emphasises the importance of whether we are able to work with others to refashion our 'habitual actions' to meet the challenge of a given situation, as a way of understanding whether an encounter supports our agency.

1.5   THE FRAGILITY OF AGENCY

Agency is *relational, constrained, situated,* and *fragile.* We may feel we are powerful agents when we have just achieved one of our goals after overcoming significant obstacles. But then our sense of agency is often compromised whenever things happen to us that we did not expect or want, as when we are victims of abuse or violence, cannot prevent the death of a loved one, or are powerless to avoid the end of a cherished relationship.

Poor mental health often undermines the feeling of agency. We may feel things that we do not understand and behave in ways that we do not recognise, when we have intense emotions or unusual experiences. Absence of empathy in the behaviour of others can 'confirm' this sense of alienation and passivity by disempowering us further (see e.g. Jackson, 2017). But others can also support us by showing us that there are steps that we can take and projects we can contribute to, even in a crisis. Those steps and those projects can be a starting point that will at some point enable us to resume a sense of worth, ownership, and (partial and temporary) control (see Pickard, 2011).

The moment when we realise that our agency is constrained and yet still valuable and needs to be cultivated and nourished like a bud in frosty weather, we can also take a kinder, more compassionate attitude to our own local failures to exercise our agency. The realisation that the people around us, and the situations we find ourselves in, shape the way we react and can support or undermine us also prompts us to work on our environment to ensure that we can identify sources of support when we need it.

We have seen in the discussion of clinical encounters, above, that we cannot always engineer the surrounding physical or social environment to our preferred specifications. It is therefore particularly important that professionals and services *designed for people experiencing mental health problems* take steps to meet us halfway. To do this, they need to provide the kinds of social relations which can support our agency and coping (through making efforts to allow us to be understood). This is especially critical when we are actively seeking help.

Acknowledgements The authors' work is supported by funding from UKRI under the MRC/AHRC/ESRC Adolescence, Mental Health and the Developing Mind: Methodological Innovation scheme for a project entitled: 'A new methodology linking interactional and experiential approaches, and involving young people as co-analysts of mental health encounters' (MR/X003108/1). Michael Larkin, Matthew Broome, Lisa Bortolotti, and Rose McCabe also acknowledge the support of project EPIC (Epistemic Injustice in Healthcare, 2023–2029), generously funded by Wellcome Discovery Award and led by Havi Carel at the University of Bristol.

REFERENCES

Anderson, C. (2022). *What to pack for psychiatric hospitalisation.* BP Hope. https://www.bphope.com/blog/what-to-pack-for-psychiatric-hospitalization/

Aoki, Y., Yaju, Y., Utsumi, T., Sanyaolu, L., Storm, M., Takaesu, Y., Watanabe, K., Watanabe, N., Duncan, E., & Edwards, A. G. K. (2022). Shared decision-making interventions for people with mental health conditions. *Cochrane Database of Systematic Reviews, 11.* Art. No.: CD007297.

Bergen, C., Bortolotti, L., Temple, R. K., Fadashe, C., Lee, C., Lim, M., McCabe, R. (2023). Implying implausibility and undermining versus accepting people's experiences of suicidal ideation and self-harm in Emergency Department psychosocial assessments. *Frontiers in Psychiatry, 14.* https://doi.org/10.3389/fpsyt.2023.1197512

Bergen, C., Bortolotti, L., Tallent, K., Broome, M., Larkin, M., Temple, R., Fadashe, C., Lee, C., Lim, M. C., & McCabe, R. (2022). Communication in youth mental health clinical encounters: Introducing the agential stance. *Theory & Psychology, 32*(5), 667–690. https://doi.org/10.1177/09593543 21095079

Bjønness S, Grønnestad T, Storm M. (2020). I'm not a diagnosis: Adolescents' perspectives on user participation and shared decision-making in mental healthcare. *Scandinavian Journal of Child and Adolescent Psychiatry and Psychology*, *8*, 139-148.https://doi.org/10.21307/sjcapp-2020-014 .

Bortolotti, L. (2013). Rationality and sanity: The role of rationality judgments in understanding psychiatric disorders. In K. W. M. Fulford et al. (Eds.), *The Oxford handbook of philosophy and psychiatry*. Oxford University Press.

Bortolotti, L., & Murphy-Hollies, K. (2023). Why we should be curious about each other. *Philosophies*, *8*(4), 71. https://doi.org/10.3390/philosophies8040071

Burkitt, I. (2018). Relational Agency. In: Dépelteau, F. (eds) *The Palgrave Handbook of Relational Sociology*. Palgrave Macmillan, Cham. https://doi.org/10.1007/978-3-319-66005-9_26

Crichton, P., Carel, H., & Kidd, I. J. (2017, April). Epistemic injustice in psychiatry. *BJPsych Bulletin*, *41*(2), 65–70. https://doi.org/10.1192/pb.bp.115.050682. PMID: 28400962; PMCID: PMC5376720. https://doi.org/10.1002/14651858.CD007297.pub3

Cruz, M., & Pincus, H. A. (2002). Research on the influence that communication in psychiatric encounters has on treatment. *Psychiatric Services.*, *53*(10), 1253–1265.

Doris, J. M. (2002). *Lack of character: Personality and moral behavior*. Cambridge University Press.

Faulkner, A. (2020). *Informing a decision guide for psychological treatments for depression: Experts by experience consultation*. National Survivor User Network. www.nsun.org.uk/resource/informing-a-decision-guide-for-psychological-treatments-for-depression

Houlders, J. W., Bortolotti, L., & Broome, M. R. (2021). Threats to epistemic agency in young people with unusual experiences and beliefs. *Synthese*, *199*(3–4), 7689–7704. https://doi.org/10.1007/s11229-021-03133-4. Epub 2021 Mar 30. PMID: 34970007; PMCID: PMC8668839.

Jackson, J. (2017). Patronizing depression: Epistemic injustice, stigmatizing attitudes, and the need for empathy. *Journal of Social Philosophy*, *48*(3), 359–376.

Kågström, A., Juríková, L., & Guerrero, Z. (2023). Developmentally appropriate mental health literacy content for school-aged children and adolescents. *Cambridge Prisms: Global Mental Health*, *10*, e25 https://doi.org/10.1017/gmh.2023.16

Kidd, I. J., Spencer, L., & Carel, H. (2022). Epistemic injustice in psychiatric research and practice. *Philosophical Psychology*, 1–29. https://doi.org/10.1080/09515089.2022.2156333

Légaré, F., Stacey, D., Turcotte, S., Cossi, M. J., Kryworuchko, J., Graham, I. D., Lyddiatt, A., Politi, M. C., Thomson, R., Elwyn, G., & Donner-Banzhoff, N. (2010). Interventions for improving the adoption of shared decision making by healthcare professionals. *Cochrane Database of Systematic Review* (5), CD006732.

Légaré, F., Turcotte, S., Stacey, D., Ratté, S., Kryworuchko, J., & Graham, I. D. (2012). Patients' perceptions of sharing in decisions: A systematic review of interventions to enhance shared decision making in routine clinical practice. *Patient, 5*, 1–19.

Maker Castro, E., Wray-Lake, L., & Cohen, A. K. (2022). Critical consciousness and wellbeing in adolescents and young adults: A systematic review. *Adolescent Research Review, 7*, 499–522. https://doi.org/10.1007/s40894-022-00188-3

McCabe, R., Bergen, C., Lomas, M., Ryan, M., & Albert, R. (2023). Asking about self-harm during risk assessment in psychosocial assessments in the emergency department: Questions that facilitate and deter disclosure of self-harm. *Bjpsych Open, 9*(3), e93. https://doi.org/10.1192/bjo.2023.32

McGorry, P. D., Mei, C., Chanen, A., Hodges, C., Alvarez-Jimenez, M., & Killackey, E. (2022). Designing and scaling up integrated youth mental health care. *World Psychiatry, 21*, 61–76. https://doi.org/10.1002/wps.20938

Nobre, J., Oliveira, A. P., Monteiro, F., Sequeira, C., & Ferré-Grau, C. (2021, September 9). Promotion of mental health literacy in adolescents: A scoping review. *International Journal of Environment Research and Public Health, 18*(18), 9500. https://doi.org/10.3390/ijerph18189500. PMID: 34574427; PMCID: PMC8470967.

Oishi, S., Koo, M., & Akimoto, S. (2008). Culture, interpersonal perceptions, and happiness in social interactions. *Personality and Social Psychology Bulletin, 34*(3), 307–320.

Oishi, S., Krochik, M., & Akimoto, S. (2010). Felt understanding as a bridge between close relationships and subjective well-being: Antecedents and consequences across individuals and cultures. *Social and Personality Psychology Compass, 4*(6), 403–416.

Patafio, B., Miller, P., Baldwin, R., Taylor, N., & Hyder, S. (2021). A systematic mapping review of interventions to improve adolescent mental health literacy, attitudes and behaviours. *Early Intervention in Psychiatry, 15*, 1470–1501. https://doi.org/10.1111/eip.13109

Pickard, H. (2011, September). Responsibility without blame: Empathy and the effective treatment of personality disorder. Philosophy, *Psychiatry, & Psychology, 18*(3), 209–223. https://doi.org/10.1353/ppp.2011.0032. PMID: 22318087; PMCID: PMC3272423.

Radez, J., Reardon, T., Creswell, C. et al. (2021). Why do children and adolescents (not) seek and access professional help for their mental health problems?

A systematic review of quantitative and qualitative studies. *European Child and Adolescent Psychiatry, 30,* 183–211. https://doi.org/10.1007/s00787-019-01469-4

Reis, H. T., Lemay, E. P., & Finkenauer, C. (2017). Toward understanding understanding: The importance of feeling understood in relationships. *Social and Personal Psychology Compass, 11,* e12308. https://doi.org/10.1111/spc3.12308

Renwick, L., Pedley, R., Johnson, I., Bell, V., Lovell, K., Bee, P., & Brooks, H. (2022). Mental health literacy in children and adolescents in low- and middle-income countries: A mixed studies systematic review and narrative synthesis. *European Child and Adolescent Psychiatry.* https://doi.org/10.1007/s00787-022-01997-6

Seedaket, S., Turnbull, N., Phajan, T., & Wanchai, A. (2020). Improving mental health literacy in adolescents: Systematic review of supporting intervention studies. *Tropical Medicine & International Health, 25,* 1055–1064. https://doi.org/10.1111/tmi.13449

Selby, C. L. B. (2019). *Therapy and counseling: Your questions answered (Q&A health guides).* Santa Barbara.

Shay, L. A., & Lafata, J. E. (2015). Where is the evidence? A systematic review of shared decision making and patient outcomes. *Medical Decision Making, 35*(1), 114–131. https://doi.org/10.1177/0272989X14551638

Slade, M. (2017). Implementing shared decision making in routine mental health care. *World Psychiatry, 16,* 146–153. https://doi.org/10.1002/wps.20412

Stone, M., Kokanovic, R., Callard, F., & Broom, A. F. (2020). Estranged relations: Coercion and care in narratives of supported decision-making in mental healthcare. *Medical Humanities, 46,* 62–72.

Strech, D., Synofzik, M., & Marckmann, G. (2008). How physicians allocate scarce resources at the bedside: A systematic review of qualitative studies. *Journal of Medicine and Philosophy, 33*(1), 80–99.

Morelli, S. A., Torre, J. B., & Eisenberger, N. I. (2014). The neural bases of feeling understood and not understood. *Social Cognitive and Affective Neuroscience, 9*(12), 1890–1896. https://doi.org/10.1093/scan/nst191

Westlund, A. (2009). Rethinking relational autonomy. *Hypatia, 24*(4), 26–49.

Williamson, V., Murphy, D., Phelps, A., Forbes, D., & Greenberg, N. (2021). Moral injury: The effect on mental health and implications for treatment. *The Lancet Psychiatry, 8*(6), 453–455.

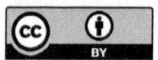

CHAPTER 2

Challenging Stereotypes About Young People Who Hear Voices

Lisa Bortolottiⓘ*, Fiona Malpass, Kathleen Murphy-Hollies*ⓘ*, Thalia Somerville-Large, Gurpriya Kapoor, and Owen Braid*

Abstract Recent work on clinical communication has highlighted the possibility that vulnerable young people may experience epistemic injustice and have their sense of agency undermined in encounters with mental healthcare providers. In particular, five dimensions of agency have been studied: validation of the person's perspective; legitimisation of the person's concerns; acknowledgement that the person may have complex interests and needs; affirmation of the person's capacity to contribute to change; and inclusion of the person in shared decision-making processes. Building on previous work in this area, and utilising the illustrative power of Aesop-style fables, we identify three potential areas where empirical investigation could help advance the study of epistemic injustice in interactions involving young people who hear voices.

L. Bortolotti (✉) · K. Murphy-Hollies
Philosophy Department and Institute for Mental Health, University of Birmingham, Birmingham, UK
e-mail: l.bortolotti@bham.ac.uk

F. Malpass · T. Somerville-Large · G. Kapoor · O. Braid
The Vioce Collective, Mind in Camden, London, UK

L. Bortolotti (ed.), *Epistemic Justice in Mental Healthcare*,
https://doi.org/10.1007/978-3-031-68881-2_2

Keywords Epistemic injustice · Hearing voices · Stereotypes · Incompetence · Dangerousness · Exclusion

2.1   STEREOTYPES

There are some common stereotypes associated with young people in our society. Young people are often thought to be lazy and immature, to lack resilience, and to be attention-seeking. For instance, they may be called "snowflakes" and "drama queens" in the press (Houlders et al., 2021). These are not just harmless stereotypes as they negatively affect the likelihood that young people are listened to with curiosity and empathy when they have something to say (Bortolotti & Murphy-Hollies, 2023).

It is not surprising then that young people's testimony about their own experiences might not be taken seriously. Their capacity to acquire and share knowledge is even more severely challenged when the mental health problems they face are particularly severe (Bergen et al., 2022), as their reports may be taken to be a product of their illness as opposed to a faithful characterisation of their experiences.

To explore these issues in the context of voice hearing, our team met to discuss the experience of young people who hear voices. Our team is composed of two academics working on agency in youth mental health, the Hearing Voices project manager, and the young people who are members of the Voice Collective. The Voice Collective is a UK-wide project that supports young people who hear voices, see visions, or have other sensory experiences or beliefs. It provides peer-support groups for anyone aged from 16 to 25.

The purpose of the team's seven meetings was to reflect on the impact of the negative stereotypes associated with young people who hear voices. As a result of the discussion during the workshop series, the team (hereafter, "we") identified a number of stereotypes that can be subsumed under the three categories of *incompetence*, *dangerousness*, and *difference leading to exclusion*. These affect the young people's interactions with the adults and peers in their lives and have the potential to cause significant harm.

In this paper, our purpose is to raise awareness of these stereotypes in the hope that we can inspire empirical work that will contribute to identify their potentially harmful consequences and propose solutions.

2.2   WHEN DISMISSING SOMEONE'S REPORT IS AN ACT OF INJUSTICE

Since ancient Greece, fables have been the means by which authors share observations and critiques of human interactions and provide recommendations about how people should behave. Typically, they are short stories with talking animals as characters and a explicit morale in the end. Consider a fable featuring a family of deer and a mountain lion, loosely inspired by the Aesop's fable entitled *The Stag and the Fawn*.

The Fawn and the Mountain Lion

In the valley, a family of deer is going to the lake to get some water before it gets dark. On the way, Fawn sees a yummy acorn stuck in the bushes and stays behind to gobble it up. Before he can eat it, though, Fawn sees Mountain Lion hiding behind a bush.

Fawn forgets all about the acorn and runs to Stag and Doe. "Mum, Dad," Fawn says, "I just saw Mountain Lion hiding behind the bushes. We have to leave, it is not safe here!"

But Stag does not appear to be worried and dismisses Fawn's warning: "Are you sure that you saw Mountain Lion? I am confident that, if Mountain Lion was nearby, I would have heard his steps. You must have imagined it."

Doe, however, looks genuinely concerned. "I think we should go back to the herd, just to be safe," she says to Stag, "Fawn has never lied to us before".

Stag is unmoved. Smiling, he asks Doe to calm down: "Don't you know that young ones can't distinguish reality from imagination? Haven't you noticed how they always try to draw attention to themselves? There is nothing to worry about here."

Then Stag invites Fawn and Doe to drink some water from the lake: "The water is fresh and delicious! Have something to drink before it gets dark. Or you will be thirsty later."

While Stag bends down to drink from the lake, Mountain Lion, who was hiding behind the bushes, leaps out and attacks him. Mountain Lion bites Stag in the leg. Luckily, before Mountain Lion can cause more damage, Owl sees what is happening from the top of a tree, and surprises Mountain Lion with loud screeches. Taken aback by the sudden noise, Mountain Lion runs away.

Owl reprimands Stag: "We sometimes dismiss a report when we don't trust the speaker due to some negative stereotype, such as the idea that young people always want to draw attention to themselves. But, in dismissing what the speaker has to say due to the stereotype, we pay a high price. We reject information that can be valuable to us."

With a sad expression, Doe adds: "You are right, wise Owl. In our herd, does and fawns are never listened to. But Fawn knows what Mountain Lion looks like! To dismiss his warning was not just risky, it was an injustice! Fawn should be taken seriously when he has something important to say.[1]

In this fable, Fawn sees Mountain Lion and warns Stag and Doe that there is danger but is not believed by his father. The reason why Fawn is not believed is important. Fawn is not known for lying, being unreliable, or seeking attention, as his mother points out. However, Stag assumes that Fawn's report is not something he should be concerned about or something that he should act upon, based on the assumption that fawns (in general) are likely to confuse reality with imagination and are attention seeking.

As the dismissal of Fawn's warning is motivated by negative stereotypes associated with the young in general, and not by a previous experience suggesting Fawn's lack of credibility, it can be construed as a case of epistemic injustice. *Epistemic injustice* occurs when an agent's perspective or report is assigned low credibility or dismissed due to a negative stereotype associated with the agent's identity (Fricker, 2007). A consequence of dismissing the agent's perspective or report may be that the agent lacks the opportunity to produce and share knowledge.

Fawn's report ("There is a mountain lion hiding in the bushes!") is dismissed due to a negative stereotype associated with aspects of Fawn's identity (in this case, being young). In the story, it is made clear that Stag's attitude is not an isolated case: Fawn's mother reflects bitterly on the fact that in a very hierarchical society like theirs, the views of fawns and does are often openly disregarded, whereas stags are taken seriously by default. What are the consequences of this?

In the fable, we see two types of effects. First, Fawn and Doe are saddened and disappointed by the fact that Stag does not take them seriously. We can imagine Fawn deciding not to warn his herd in the future for fear of being ignored and ridiculed. Second, after ignoring Fawn's

---

[1] *The Fawn and the Mountain Lion* is also a short animated video that can be found here: https://youtu.be/WrD-4UkPijo?si=pmvYzwjGZq3kVbE6. It was produced by Squideo on the basis of a script written by Lisa Bortolotti to illustrate the notion of epistemic injustice.

warning, Stag is attacked and wounded by Mountain Lion, who runs away only when Owl screeches loudly, causing a commotion. The fact that Stag ignores Fawn's warning causes harm to Fawn who does not get the opportunity to share knowledge and contribute to collective decision making. But it also causes harm to Stag himself who cannot rely on important information that could be used to prevent the attack.

From the point of view of young people who hear voices, dismissing the perspectives of the vulnerable, or of those who hold less power in a relationship, has harmful consequences that are pervasive and lasting: even reacting against that dismissal can become ineffectual in some contexts where the stereotypes are widely accepted and go unchallenged. Commenting on the video of *The Fawn and the Mountain Lion*, one of the young people said:

> Often there is not really any material harm at all to the powerful person who dismisses the perspective of the vulnerable person. Often even more harm is done to vulnerable people who try to hold powerful people to account via formal channels which also hold power and can repeat the original scenario by dismissing the vulnerable person's perspective again. This leaves the person in power with the ability to go on dismissing more vulnerable people over and over, often with no repercussion whatsoever.

In an alternative version of the fable where Stag does not get attacked by Mountain Lion in the end, we can imagine further harm coming to fawns and does, despite their warnings and pleas for help, whilst stags carry on blissfully unaware.

Fables are by nature short and there is a limit to the complexity of the situations they can shed light on. Typically, there is no room to explore the consequences of the event being narrated and there is no long-term character development in the fable itself. However, *The Fawn and the Mountain Lion* shows some interesting features of epistemic injustice, including the pervasive and harmful nature of unquestioned stereotypes and the fact that such stereotypes harm the vulnerable person whose report is dismissed but also (in a different way and possibly to a lesser extent) the powerful person who dismisses it.

2.3   WHEN STEREOTYPES ABOUT YOUNG PEOPLE WHO HEAR VOICES CAUSE HARM

In our team, we decided to write a new fable exploring instances of epistemic injustice and their consequences for young people who hear voices. Structurally, the story is similar to the one discussed in the previous section, as it is a short story based on the interaction amongst animal characters with a explicit message in the end. However, for this fable, our focus was narrower. We wanted to explore how some of the widespread assumptions about young people who hear voices compromise their capacity to exercise agency and the quality of their social relationships.

As explained in a classic paper on mental health stigma (Corrigan & Watson, 2002), the results of extensive public surveys in the Western, anglophone world suggest that there are three prevalent stereotypes associated with people with poor mental health: they are to be feared, and thus excluded; they are irresponsible, so they are unable to make decisions for themselves; and they are "childlike," so they need to be taken care of. These stereotypes concern people's agency, that is, their capacity to intervene in the world around them and pursue their goals based on their beliefs, intentions, desires, and values. If people with poor mental health are described as dangerous, irresponsible, and childlike, this suggests that they are not seen as agents.

Young people who hear voices and have other unusual experiences and beliefs tend to be seen as seriously ill and, thus, dangerous to themselves and others. Moreover, their capacity to exercise agency and act autonomously is regarded as so severely compromised that social interactions with them are thought to be unproductive, leading to exclusion. One common observation is that, when these assumptions take hold, they are difficult to dislodge, even when young people no longer behave in ways that are taken to confirm them.

Here is the fable we produced in our team, representing the potential harms of negative stereotypes about young people who hear voices, which we entitled *The Wolf, the Snake, and the Butterfly*.

The Wolf, the Snake, and the Butterfly

Wolf, Snake, and Butterfly meet in the clearing. Butterfly is surprised to see Wolf: "Wolf, what are you doing here?" Butterfly asks, "Hasn't your pack moved on last night?" With a sad expression on his face, Wolf replies: "They left at sunset without me... with my limp they think I'll be a burden."

Snake is also surprised to see Butterfly in the clearing where there are hardly any flowers: "Butterfly, what are you doing in the clearing?" Snake asks, "Isn't the poppy field more your scene?". Shaking her head, Butterfly replies: "Well, the poppy field is lovely but I'm tired of the teasing. Bee keeps saying that I don't pull my weight." Snake cannot believe it: "What nonsense! Without your constant wandering, there would be hardly any poppies!" Butterfly agrees that she is a good pollinator now. But she explains that in the past she was not: "When I was a caterpillar, Bee saw me eating all day long. Bee will always see me as the useless one..."

Snake nods and adds: "Stereotypes are hard to overcome. I'm really gentle, but humans run scared when they see me and even beat me with a stick if they get the chance!" Wolf joins in: "Ah, snakes and wolves win no popularity contest! Aren't we always the villains in fairy tales?"

Wolf, Snake and Butterfly compare their experiences to those of young people who hear voices.

Wolf reflects on the problem of difference leading to exclusion: "We're often isolated because we're different, as the boy in the playground who is told that he makes his friends uncomfortable, and they no longer want to play with him."

Snake reflects on the stereotype of dangerousness: "Even those who are there to support us consider us dangerous, as the doctor who tells a young patient in the clinic that she does not feel safe in a room alone with her, and is going to ask a colleague to join them."

Butterfly reflects on the stereotype of incompetence: "We are treated as if we can't achieve anything, as the student who is advised to withdraw from the programme by his university lecturer because people who hear voices are too unwell to cope."

Snake concludes: "When others find us useless or dangerous, or exclude us because we are different, we experience harm and it's harder for us to do the things that we value." And Butterfly adds: "But we have a lot to offer!"[2]

Both our group discussions and the work on the fable *The Wolf, the Snake, and the Butterfly* were inspired by recent attempts in philosophy

---

[2] *The Wolf, the Snake, and the Butterfly* is also a short animated video that can be found here: https://youtu.be/c1uAqpI-Hjo. It was produced by Squideo on the basis of a script written by our team, which includes members of the Voice Collective. It is meant to illustrate the potential harm of negative stereotypes associated with young people who hear voices.

to think about the effects of interpersonal relationships on agency in the context of mental health. As it has been shown in previous work (Sakakibara, 2023; Sanati & Kyratsous, 2015), the question whether people experience epistemic injustice seems to be especially relevant for people who access psychiatric services for serious illness, as their capacity for rational thought and autonomous decision making are often assumed to be compromised by their struggles with mental health issues (Kidd et al., 2022; Ritunnano, 2022).

More specifically, our team reflected on the consequences of stereotypes on the capacity of young people who hear voices to exercise agency. Based on the young people's experiences, we started discussing whether hearing voices makes people vulnerable to negative stereotypes and then we moved on to think about the potential effects of those stereotypes. The fable aims to draw attention to the circumstances in which young people who hear voices are made to feel *excluded because different* (Wolf), *incompetent* or *useless* (Butterfly), and *dangerous* (Snake). Not all instances of stereotyping amount to epistemic injustice but acting on the misconceptions we identified can be a form of epistemic injustice when young people are denied credibility and agency merely because they hear voices.

Due to their occasionally departing from consensual reality, people who hear voices are not thought to be in a position to share knowledge, engage in decision making, and contribute to positive change in their lives. Individual and collective attitudes towards young people who hear voices, in peer groups, the family, the school environment, and also in the healthcare system, imply that their capacity to exercise agency is compromised. Unfortunately, this occurs even when the young people do demonstrate awareness that their own experiences may differ from the experiences of others and actively seek help and take the initiative in their care.

It is not difficult to see how a person's young age combined with behaviours that are characterised as symptoms of psychosis can give rise to negative stereotypes. As mentioned in the previous section, common misconceptions about young people include that they are immature and reckless, lack resilience, and crave attention. To these, we can add the widespread belief that people who struggle with their mental health are irrational and unable to identify and pursue their best interests—especially when they report unusual experiences and beliefs, and do not share the same view of reality as those around them.

In recent empirical work with young people who struggle with their mood and have suicidal thoughts (Bergen et al., 2022), the authors suggested that healthcare practitioners could adopt an *agential stance* during emergency assessments in order to protect and enhance the young people's capacity to exercise their agency, whilst acknowledging that young people accessing emergency services may be experiencing a crisis and need support. Five steps to sustain agency were identified: (1) validating the young person's experience; (2) recognising that the young person has legitimate concerns that should be addressed; (3) avoiding the practice of diagnostically labelling the young person prematurely, before considering their perspective and situation; (4) affirming the young person's capacity to contribute to positive change; and (5) involving the young person in the decision-making process.

Although these five areas are likely to be relevant to the protection of agency in other vulnerable populations as well (Bortolotti, 2023, Chapter 8), there are important differences in how agency is threatened depending on the specific nature of the vulnerability identified in the agents and the negative stereotypes those vulnerabilities trigger. For instance, when talking to young people struggling with their mood, it is not uncommon to hear that practitioners challenge the young people's description of their own feelings and suggest that involving emergency services might have been unnecessary. This leads to the sense that the young people's concerns were not legitimate to start with (see Bergen et al., 2023 for some examples).

However, for young people who hear voices and have other unusual experiences and beliefs, this is a much less pressing issue because their behaviours are regarded as symptomatic of severe distress and thus their concerns are more likely to be taken seriously (often too seriously, as we shall see) by practitioners. Other potential threats to agency are more prominent in the case of young people hearing voices, including the fact that young people are regarded as potentially dangerous to themselves and others, and as lacking capacity altogether. The young people's lack of capacity may be considered so significant that their potential for bringing about positive change and for contributing to decision making is ruled out entirely.

One point often raised in our discussions was that, in interactions with practitioners, young people found very little acknowledgement of the fact that voice hearing can be a positive thing (Parry & Varese, 2021). Some young people find some of their voices comforting but this is not some-thing explicitly acknowledged in clinical encounters: as one young person put it, "voice hearing is always taken as a threat that needs to be fixed, further invalidating our experiences."

This speaks to the risks of objectification: in interactions with others in general, and in the healthcare context in particular, the person in a position to provide support sometimes sees the other as a problem to be fixed rather than as a complex agent with multiple needs and interests. The voices may be seen "just as a problem," for instance, rather than "a problem and also a coping mechanism that offers comfort."

2.4   THREE STEREOTYPES

2.4.1   *Butterfly, or Misattributions of Incompetence*

In the fable, Butterfly is regarded as "useless" by Bee because, at the stage of being a caterpillar, she did not contribute to pollination and instead was seen eating all day long. It is of course necessary for caterpillars to eat as much as they can, so they acquire the right size to go into the pupal stage. This means that there is nothing "useless" about the caterpillar feeding, and we know that caterpillars make a number of important contributions to their ecosystems as well. For instance, they prevent vegetation from growing too quickly and depleting nutrients in the soil.

But we can also understand how, from Bee's perspective, caterpil-lars may not appear to contribute as much as bees to the life of the garden. However, caterpillars turn into butterflies, and butterflies are excellent pollinators, as is acknowledged in the fable. So, Caterpillar being described as useless by Bee is an understandable misconception, but Butterfly being described as useless suggests that a negative judgement that might have been understandable in the past, though not justified, has not shifted and is now entirely inappropriate.

How does Butterfly's story relate to the experiences of young people who hear voices? One of the young people explains:

> We picked a caterpillar transitioning into a butterfly to represent how assumptions can still apply to voice hearers no matter their current circum-stance and if they are not in crisis. In the video, Caterpillar is assumed to be useless by Bee as it is only eating so it can grow to become a butterfly and once it becomes a butterfly it is still assumed to be useless even though it is now pollinating the flowers. This reflects how voice hearers can be

perceived as lacking capacity to do things, such as being asked to with-draw from programmes in higher education just because they hear voices. We wanted to represent how these assumptions are not reflective of voice hearers and that they are still capable even though they hear voices. We wanted to represent how voice hearers are not defined by the fact that they hear voices and their conditions.

One aspect that is worth exploring is the fact that a judgement that is made at some point in the past about the unusual behaviour of young people who hear voices can often be made again and again, even when young people no longer engage in those behaviours. As young people who hear voices observed, the presence of one instance of voice hearing or of an unusual belief is often sufficient to wipe out the perceived autonomy of the young person altogether, and for a very long time: "If you have a delusion once, then everything you do is interpreted in the light of it. You are always seen as lacking capacity." One example of this is when being non-compliant with medication or seeing things differently from the healthcare practitioner is considered as a sign of illness and as evidence that the young person lacks capacity. The risk is that concerns with medication or other forms of treatment may not be addressed.

Diagnostic labels may also persist although people's experiences evolve and change. One experience that seems to be common to young people who hear voices is that they are assigned a diagnostic label early on, when they first access services, often after a superficial exploration of their experiences and concerns. Although the label is not explained or discussed with the young person in detail, it affects all future interactions with healthcare professionals because it remains in their medical notes.

2.4.2   Snake, or Misattributions of Dangerousness

In the fable, Snake is regarded as "dangerous" by the humans who cross his path. We know there is a strong association in popular culture between snakes and evil, starting from the biblical story in the garden of Eden up to the Harry Potter books where snakes are natural allies to Lord Voldemort. Given the bad press snakes get, it is not surprising that people fear snakes. But it is a misconception that all or most snakes are aggressive and poisonous. Not all snakes release toxins when they bite (in the UK, for instance, only the adder is poisonous). And snakes are almost never aggressive towards humans: they may react if we try to pick them up but in most cases the reaction consists in crawling away.

How does Snake's story relate to the experiences of young people who hear voices? The first observation to make is that the experience of voice hearing is not the same for everyone and can also present different characteristics and be more or less significant for the same individual at different times. The heterogeneity that is explored in recent phenomenological analyses of the experience of voice hearing (Woods et al., 2015) needs to be acknowledged.

In clinical encounters, it was observed that some behaviours, interpreted as symptoms of severe distress, may be taken *too seriously* in the sense that they overshadow other problems that the young person is experiencing and that may be more important to them at the time. For instance, one young person said: "I feel that anxiety is a more pressing problem than hearing voices for me now, but anxiety is systematically downplayed by others as all their attention is devoted to my voices."

Hearing voices and having unusual beliefs are often associated with dangerousness, and thus young people who hear voices are sometimes treated as if they were a threat to the safety of others, even when there is no indication or evidence that this is the case. As one of the young people put it, this misconception of dangerousness "can cause overreactions that lead professionals to involve emergency services even when no actual immediate risk is present, without the person's consent. This can often put that person in the way of further harm as emergency services often escalate a situation and can cause more trauma to the vulnerable person."

Interestingly, a connection can be drawn between misconceptions of dangerousness and the superficiality with which the experiences of young people who hear voices are sometimes addressed in clinical encounters and elsewhere. When the experiences are underexplored, there is a greater risk that they may be misunderstood. Especially the experiences and behaviours considered to be a serious threat to agency may not be thoroughly investigated by practitioners. As one of the young people put it: "As they did not ask me questions about my experience, I had no opportunity to share how I was feeling, and they misunderstood what my experience was."

2.4.3 Wolf, or the Problem of Difference Leading to Exclusion

In the fable, Wolf is different from the other wolves in his pack. He has a small injury in his leg, and this makes the rest of the pack think that he will be a burden when they move to a new territory, because the assumption is that he won't be running as fast, and he won't be as successful as a hunter. So, Wolf is left behind. Wolves are highly intelligent and sociable animals, capable of developing strong bonds with members of their packs. Being left behind in the way Wolf is in the fable would be a big deal and being isolated or excluded can be very distressing.

As well as having to cope with exclusion due to being different, Wolf experiences the effects of negative stereotypes, just like Butterfly and Snake. Like Butterfly, he is thought to be useless. But there is no good reason to believe that a small injury (which is likely to heal) will prevent Wolf from contributing to the life of the pack. Like Snake, Wolf suffers from a bad reputation: snakes may be routinely associated with evil, but wolves are the default villains in fairy tales, eating helpless old ladies and chasing cute little pigs. Yet, in real life, wolves very rarely attack humans and can form lasting bonds with them.

How does Wolf's story relate to the experiences of young people who hear voices? The experience of exclusion due to perceived dangerousness, uselessness, or merely illness was reported consistently by young people who described interactions with peers, teachers, and healthcare professionals as alienating. This interesting phenomenon was characterised as a catch-22: if young people are seen as capable of articulating the reasons for their own distress in the clinical encounter, and participate in decision making, then they are often deemed "not ill enough" to be worthy of additional support, or they are seen as "being manipulative" or "playing the system." But if young people are seen as incapable of acknowledging the extent of their own distress and lacking the capacity to contribute to positive change, then they are straight-forwardly excluded from conversations and decisions about their future—for instance, the practitioner may address the parents and not the young person, talking about the young person as if they were not present. Both situations bring about forms of exclusion: if the young person is seen as capable but manipulative, they are excluded from decision making because they do not have the right intentions; if the young person is seen as sincere but incapacitated, they are excluded from decision making because they cannot make a meaningful contribution.

As one young person said:

As someone who hears voices and has unusual experiences, healthcare settings feel deeply unsafe. Every time I interact with medical professionals there is a danger that they will decide that I am either lacking in capacity or a manipulative and 'difficult' patient. These decisions are then written into medical records that will follow me for years (regardless of whether the professional's original judgements were made with bias are no longer relevant today). The effects of removing someone's agency reach far beyond a single (often brief) interaction and continue to harm a patient years into the future.

One general problem which applies to agency in a number of different contexts is that often capacity is seen as an all-or-nothing property of the person and there is little recognition that some people can contribute to some projects and fail to contribute to other projects. As one young person put it, "If I demonstrate agency in one dimension of my life, people then insist that I exercise agency over other behaviours over which I may not have full control."

Young people who hear voices often found that decisions were made on their behalf about what they were capable of. Sometimes young people felt more capable than it was perceived by others. When facing challenging projects, the decision was to exclude them whereas they felt that that they would have been able to participate with some additional support. In the fable, we see how the university lecturer advises the young man to withdraw from the programme instead of offering further support. There is an element of self-fulfilling prophecy there—it is because young people who hear voices are excluded that they are often perceived as "lone wolves."

Another related problem is that we tend to see agency as tied to praise and blame, and thus we associate attributions of agency with attributions of responsibility. If a person is thought to be capable of acting on their best interests and participating in decision making, then they are also expected to take responsibility for the outcome of their actions and the consequences of the decisions they contribute to make. However, agency does not imply infallibility, omnipotence, or even control over external circumstances.

Human agents are *imperfect agents* because they always make decisions in situations of uncertainty and do not have complete knowledge of all the relevant variables. They are always *situated agents* because they are constrained in what they do by their physical and social environment. In other words, their agency can be supported or hindered by a number of factors, including the attitudes of the people around them (Bortolotti, 2020, Chapters 1 and 7). In situations of crisis, attributing the capacity to contribute to change to the person in distress may be helpful if it is accompanied by adequate support, but praising or blaming may be unhelpful as it can put a lot of pressure on the person whose actions and decisions are scrutinised (Brandenburg, 2017; Pickard, 2013). That is why, in formulating the agential stance, it is preferable to talk about the capacity to contribute to change as a more feasible and less demanding attribute of agency than full responsibility over actions and decisions.

However, in many social interactions, adults in position of authority routinely challenge the capacity of young people who hear voices and are also quick to adopt a judgemental approach, holding young people responsible for behaviours that are perceived as problematic, such as not complying with medication or self-harming. The attribution of responsibility in these contexts fails to take into account the situatedness of agency and the multiple factors that may give rise to the problematic behaviours, and is rarely accompanied by a genuine attempt to understand the reasons behind those behaviours.

2.5   Inspiring Research and Changing Practice

In this paper, we used the means of an Aesop-style fable to illustrate some of the experiences of young people who hear voices. Our goal was to reflect on the potential harms of negative stereotypes, inspired by philosophical literature on epistemic injustice in mental health and by the lived experience of the members of the Voice Collective.

We focused on the impact of such stereotypes on the capacity of young people to exercise their agency and contribute to shared epistemic projects. We hope that the three broad areas we identified (incompetence, dangerousness, and difference leading to exclusion) can be the object of empirical work on potential epistemic injustice in education and healthcare settings and that the findings will help support concrete suggestions to alleviate the effects of stereotypes associated with young people who hear voices.

Acknowledgements Work on this chapter was possible thanks to support from Mind in Camden, the Voice Collective, and EPIC (Epistemic Injustice in Healthcare, 2023–2029), a project generously funded by a Wellcome Discovery Award and led by Havi Carel at the University of Bristol. We thank Shioma-Lei Craythorne for useful comments on a previous version of this chapter.

REFERENCES

Aesop. (1881). *Aesop's Fables*. W.M.L. Allison.

Brandenburg, D. (2017). The nurturing stance: Making sense of responsibility without blame. *Pacific Philosophical Quarterly, 99*(S1), 5–22.

Bortolotti, L. (2023). *Why delusions matter*. Bloomsbury.

Bortolotti, L. (2020). *The epistemic innocence of irrational beliefs*. Oxford University Press.

Bortolotti, L., & Murphy-Hollies, K. (2023). Why we should be curious about each other. *Philosophies, 8*(4), 71. https://doi.org/10.3390/philosophies8040071

Bergen, C., Bortolotti, L., Tallent, K., Broome, M., Larkin, M., Temple, R., Fadashe, C., Lee, C., Lim, M. C., & McCabe, R. (2022). Communication in youth mental health clinical encounters: Introducing the agential stance. *Theory & Psychology, 32*(5), 667–690. https://doi.org/10.1177/09593543221095079

Bergen, C., Bortolotti, L., Temple, R. K., Fadashe, C., Lee, C., Lim, M., & McCabe, R. (2023). Implying implausibility and undermining versus accepting peoples' experiences of suicidal ideation and self-harm in Emergency Department psychosocial assessments. *Frontiers in Psychiatry, 14*. https://doi.org/10.3389/fpsyt.2023.1197512

Corrigan, P. W., & Watson, A. C. (2002). Understanding the impact of stigma on people with mental illness. *World Psychiatry (WPA), 1*(1), 16–20.

Fricker, M. (2007). *Epistemic injustice: Power and the ethics of knowing*. Oxford University Press.

Houlders, J. W., Bortolotti, L., & Broome, M. R. (2021). Threats to epistemic agency in young people with unusual experiences and beliefs. *Synthese, 199*, 7689–7704. https://doi.org/10.1007/s11229-021-03133-4

Kidd, I. J., Spencer, L., & Carel, H. (2022). Epistemic injustice in psychiatric research and practice. *Philosophical Psychology*. https://doi.org/10.1080/09515089.2022.2156333

Parry, S., & Varese, F. (2021). Whispers, echoes, friends and fears: Forms and functions of voice-hearing in adolescence. *Child Adolescent Mental Health, 26*, 195–203. https://doi.org/10.1111/camh.12403

Ritunnano, R. (2022). Overcoming hermeneutical injustice in mental health: A role for critical phenomenology. *Journal of the British Society for Phenomenology*, *53*(3), 1–18. https://doi.org/10.1080/00071773.2022.203 1234

Pickard, H. (2013). Responsibility without blame: Philosophical reflections on clinical practice. In B. Fulford, M. Davies, R. Gipps, G. Graham, J. Sadler, G. Stanghellini, & T. Thornton (Eds.), *The Oxford handbook of philosophy and psychiatry* (pp. 1134–1152). Oxford University Press.

Sakakibara, E. (2023). Epistemic injustice in the therapeutic relationship in psychiatry. *Theoretical Medicine and Bioethics*, *44*(5), 477–502. https://doi.org/10.1007/s11017-023-09627-1

Sanati, A., & Kyratsous, M. (2015). Epistemic injustice in assessment of delusions. *Journal of Evaluation in Clinical Practice*, *21*(3), 479–485. https://doi.org/10.1111/jep.12347

Woods, A., Jones, N., Alderson-Day, B., Callard, F., & Fernyhough, C. (2015). Experiences of hearing voices: Analysis of a novel phenomenological survey. *The Lancet Psychiatry*, *2*(4), 323–331. https://doi.org/10.1016/S2215-036 6(15)00006-1

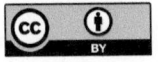

Reacting to Demoralization and Investigating the Experience of Dignity in Psychosis: Reflections from an Acute Psychiatric Ward

Martino Belvederi Murri◉, Federica Folesani◉,
Maria Giulia Nanni◉, and Luigi Grassi◉

Abstract Psychotic disorders are extremely challenging for individuals and their loved ones. The experience of psychosis, as is found in schizophrenia, may subvert the foundations of the individual's relationship with the world. Irrespective of the theoretical frame of reference, psychotic episodes are characterized by intrinsic impairment of the individual ability to know, make sense of, and experience the world, thus limiting agency and threatening dignity. In addition, individuals with acute psychosis are generally cared for within institutions that entail some degree of separation from society (e.g. the psychiatric ward) and—in extreme cases—with coercive practices. Coercion is established by the

M. Belvederi Murri (✉) · F. Folesani · M. G. Nanni · L. Grassi
Institute of Psychiatry, Department of Neuroscience and Rehabilitation,
University of Ferrara, Ferrara, Italy
e-mail: martino.belvederimurri@unife.it

© The Author(s) 2025
L. Bortolotti (ed.), *Epistemic Justice in Mental Healthcare*,
https://doi.org/10.1007/978-3-031-68881-2_3

law as a "necessary evil" to avoid risky outcomes and to achieve clinical improvements, i.e. recover a better contact with reality. However, this approach may engender situations that are detrimental for individual dignity, morale, and epistemic justice. During the emergence of acute severe mental illness and its treatment, individuals may in fact encounter stigmatization and marginalization, and experience stress, loss of agency and loss of dignity. After one or more hospital admissions, the experience of severe mental illness and the conditions related to treatment may engender demoralization, which is particularly detrimental in the long term and may increase the risk of suicide. This chapter aims to provide an overview of the available evidence on these topics and broad indications on strategies and .therapeutic approaches that might improve the experience of psychiatric inpatient care.

Keywords Psychosis · Schizophrenia · Acute ward · Epistemic justice · Dignity · Coercion · Marginalization

3.1   PSYCHOSIS, INSIGHT, AND CAPACITY

This chapter discusses the unique challenges faced by individuals experiencing acute psychosis treated within the inpatient psychiatric settings. We discuss how patient symptoms, lack of insight, and unwillingness to receive care may lead to involuntary treatment, the last resource to address the potential risks in such clinical situations. Coercive treatment, however, poses significant threats to agency and epistemic justice. Against the backdrop of evolving principles of care, but pressing resource constraints, we pursue an examination of how aspects related both to psychosis and coercive practices may lead to the erosion of dignity, agency, and morale during inpatient treatment. Despite the scarcity of literature addressing these topics, we focus on elucidating the complex issues arising when psychosis and/or its management endanger patient agency and epistemic justice, and what principles and initiatives may be considered to reduce this burden.

Psychosis entails a disruption in the individual's perception of reality. Psychotic disorders are characterized by symptoms such as hallucinations, delusions, disorganized thinking, and significant social or occupational dysfunction. This group of conditions not only affects the individual's internal world but also their interactions with the external environment, leading to profound challenges in understanding and navigating the social, occupational, and existential aspects of their lives. The complexity of psychotic disorders lies both in their postulated causes and their kaleidoscopic manifestations, ranging from acute episodes of schizophrenia to the mood-congruent psychotic features of bipolar disorder. Each variant of psychosis presents unique challenges, requiring a nuanced approach to treatment (Kuipers et al., 2014).

The symptoms of psychosis often emerge in late adolescence or early adulthood, marking a delicate period of transition and development, when existential crises are nearly physiological. They may aggravate an already challenged sense of reality and self-identity, which becomes even more fragmented and uncertain (Lysaker & Lysaker, 2010). The manifestations of psychosis vary widely amongst individuals, but may fundamentally alter one's perception, emotion, and understanding of the world. Consider the case of Jake, a student who is struggling between familial conflicts and economic difficulties, as well as choices related to his career. Auditory hallucinations may take the form of "voices" that comment on everyday actions, and may lead Jake to think that people spy on him with malevolent intent. These symptoms can lead to angst and withdrawal from social activities, possibly culminating into severe anxiety and agitation. In similar cases, violent behaviour may also be present, although it is rare. The belief in the realness of voices and persecution exemplifies the convincing nature of psychotic symptoms (Belvederi Murri et al., 2021a). The onset of psychosis can be sudden or quite gradual, and may be preceded by other experiences with core existential themes including loss of common sense, perplexity, and lack of immersion in the world with compromised vital contact with reality, perturbation of the sense of self, and need to hide tumultuous inner experiences. In the first episode, the acute phase is denoted by intense self-referentiality and permeated self-world boundaries and dissolution of the sense of self (Fusar-Poli et al., 2022).

It is not surprising that acute psychosis is often accompanied by the lack of awareness that such experience constitutes an illness and deserves treatment. In other words, individuals often lack insight into their condition (Belvederi Murri & Amore, 2018; David, 1990; Henriksen & Parnas, 2014). Education, cultural factors, and societal attitudes towards mental health can profoundly affect how a person internalizes and acknowledges their mental health conditions (Kirmayer & Looper, 2006). The grave societal stigma that is attached to mental illness (Foucault et al., 2013) exacerbates individual feelings of isolation and diminishes help-seeking (Clement et al., 2015). In these cases, decision-making capacity needs to be carefully assessed. Clinicians are called upon to explore patients' reasoning in detail, facilitating more meaningful discussions around treatment decisions (David, 2020). This aspect is crucial to determine the degree of patient autonomy and involvement in healthcare decisions, strictly intertwined with agency, human dignity, and rights. The promotion of patient empowerment is a key component of recovery, and is increasingly seen as a duty of healthcare providers (Larkin & Hutton, 2017). Pertinent themes include a desire for respect and understanding by healthcare providers, the need for clear and empathetic communication, and genuine involvement in decision-making (Stovell et al., 2016).

3.2   Treatment of Psychosis Within Inpatient Settings

The treatment of psychosis has evolved significantly, with current clinical guidelines advocating for a comprehensive, multidisciplinary approach (Maj et al., 2021). Treatment encompasses a range of pharmacological, psychological, and supportive interventions. Antipsychotic medications are one cornerstone of treatment, and reduce the severity of hallucinations and delusions. However, medication alone is insufficient. Psychotherapy, social support, and rehabilitation programs mark the shift towards a person- and recovery-centred approach. Early intervention services are particularly important to support the individual since the initial stages of psychotic experiences, and also address the broader impact psychosis has on education, employment, and social relationships, ultimately improving long-term outcomes (Belvederi Murri et al., 2021b, 2023). However, such a focus on empowerment, identity, meaning, and resilience is not always ensured in ordinary clinical practice (Maj et al., 2021).

3.2.1   Coercive Practices: Necessities and Implications

Enabling human rights and deinstitutionalization are fundamental priorities for Mental Health in the twenty-first century; coercive practices are in stark contrast with such basic human rights, at least apparently. In fact, it is purely ideological and hypocritical to deny that psychosis *can* entail situations where there is grave danger for the person and/or other people, and where decision-making capacity is severely impaired (Walsh et al., 2002).

In exemplary cases, suicidal or violent behaviour is a danger requiring immediate action. In some cases, only coercive interventions can prevent harm or severe damage to people. In such cases, the law *authorizes* or, better, *prescribes* coercive treatment modalities in various forms (Burns et al., 2016; Zaami et al., 2020). Coercive inpatient treatment in psychiatric settings may take the modality of Community Treatment Orders, forced treatment, involuntary admissions, seclusion and restriction, and informal coercion (Aragonés-Calleja & Sánchez-Martínez, 2024).

Seclusion into "locked wards" or "alienation" from society is one of the most common coercive practices in the history of humankind (Foucault et al., 2013). From a historical perspective, we actually witness the infancy stage of community-based, recovery-oriented psychiatry (Badano, 2024). Seclusion has broad-ranging ethical and medico-legal implications (Zaami et al., 2020). In high-income countries, the debate mainly regards the contrast between "open door" policies vs. "locked door" practices, but it is not yet informed by robust evidence (Beaglehole et al., 2017). Research intuitively indicates that patients often report extremely negative psychological effects of seclusion, including feelings of confinement and frustration. Patient and ward characteristics, however, only partially explain the variations in seclusion practices. Ward policies, the level of staffing and other contingencies may play a decisive role in the frequency of seclusion. This highlights the need for thoughtful policy-making and adequate resources to minimize seclusion (Gooding et al., 2020).

Forced medication is also a dramatically common, particularly with schizophrenia and other psychotic disorders, when there has been violent behaviour. This approach is aimed at managing immediate risks but raises significant ethical concerns. Available research leaves uncertainty concerning the implications and effectiveness of such practices (Jarrett et al., 2008).

Another issue is informal coercion, i.e. a spectrum of strategies like persuasion, leverage, and inducement to influence patient decisions regarding treatment. These methods may be employed by mental health professionals and staff to enhance adherence to general rules, treatment plans and improve overall health outcomes. Such strategies haunt the ethical landscape by potentially compromising patient autonomy and dignity but persist because they are considered effective in achieving clinical goals and may prevent formal coercion. Ethical debates focus on the balance between beneficial outcomes and methods to achieve them, highlighting the need for clear guidelines and transparent practices (Valenti et al., 2015). A recent qualitative study on informal coercion in psychiatry highlighted relative themes amongst mental health professionals: there is a universal belief in its effectiveness, particularly for enhancing treatment adherence, but this is accompanied by "ethical discomfort" about employing it. Finally, the underlying conflict between paternalism and the respect for patient autonomy frames the ethical landscape (Valenti et al., 2015).

3.2.2   *The Impact of Coercive Practices on Patients and Staff: A Matter of Agency and Dignity*

To provide an overview of the implications of coercive measures, we limit the discussion to cases where coercion is applied *appropriately*, lawfully, and ethically (Hoff, 2015). In such cases, admission and treatment are highly recommended and *constitute themselves the core of dignified care*. It is difficult to demonstrate it, but it should be stressed that coercion and involuntary admissions can have positive consequences and may even save lives. Since early intervention is universally recommended in psychosis, another argument in favour of coercive admission is that it reduces the latency of treatment (duration of untreated psychosis), a risk factor for future chronicization of delusions, and other manifestations of psychosis (Large et al., 2008). The other argument relies on the fact that involuntary admissions are generally used in case of suicide risk, violent behaviour or risk for others, neglect and poor self-care, behaviours that threaten dignity and are harmful for the individual aspirations related to their professional and social life. These conditions are relatively common. With hindsight, some individuals who were treated compulsorily considered the experience as a "*necessary emergency brake*" (Sibitz et al., 2011) to protect them against their own behaviours, which they judged subsequently against their own best interest (Lorem et al., 2015).

Similarly, some users report a paradoxical sense of safety in isolation, appreciating the protective aspect despite the overarching negative impact of seclusion (Aragonés-Calleja & Sánchez-Martínez, 2024; Douglas et al., 2022). In another study, the vast majority of acutely admitted patients were satisfied with treatment, with little differences between those admitted involuntarily and voluntarily, except for their satisfaction with the information provided to them. The provision of sufficient and adequate information even during coercive measures is an important target for mental healthcare service improvement (Bø et al., 2016).

There is a dearth of recommendations guiding care within coercive conditions; the call for guidelines is imperative (Maiese et al., 2019; NICE guidance, 2018). The "principle of least coercive care", however, has been proposed to limit the extent of these practices to the minimal necessary intervention. Clearly, coercion should only be considered empirically justified if the client is incompetent *in that situation* and the harm caused by coercion is significantly less than the harm that would occur if the client were left uncoerced (O'Brien & Golding, 2003).

This approach challenges traditional views and calls for a careful assessment of how coercive a practice is, which can vary significantly from case to case. However, a general ranking of coercive practices was proposed to provide guidance, illustrating a continuum from overt force to subtle influences that respect client autonomy (O'Brien & Golding, 2003). The application in the real world, however, seems still heterogeneous at best (Dutra et al., 2022). At present, available data suggest that there may be bias towards more frequent application of coercion depending on the individual's ethnicity, gender, and culture (Isohanni et al., 1991; Keane et al., 2019; Knight et al., 2022; Witt et al., 2013).

Lastly, even when coercion is applied appropriately, it may profoundly impact the individual dignity and sense of agency. For instance, when a patient needs mechanical restraint or seclusion due to aggressiveness, even when the necessary measures are taken (provide information, offer fluids and food, pay attention, attempt to understand why the patient acted that way) they may view this as a violation of human rights or as punishment, and have a painful traumatic experience (Dutra et al., 2022). Between these measures, the seclusion room is generally considered less detrimental (Huf et al., 2012). Patients may be sidelined in decisions about their care, humiliated, de-humanized, and discriminated.

In the long term, coercion may diminish their autonomy and control over their treatment and recovery process beyond what is strictly necessary. This loss of agency may also challenge the very foundation of their identity and self-worth. Those who were subject to coercive practices described feeling imprisoned and dehumanized, particularly when subjected to restrictive measures like seclusion or involuntary admission. Psychological distress or even trauma are reported in up to 70% of cases (Guzmán-Parra et al., 2019).

The theme of dignity is still generally understudied. Core themes that emerge in inpatient treatment are those of powerlessness, quality of care environment, relationship to staff, psychological and physical impact of involuntary treatment, and paradoxes (Plunkett & Kelly, 2021; Plunkett et al., 2022). Patients frequently described experience of coercive practices as aversive, but some also perceived that some level of coercion was necessary. Conflicting views were also reported on "house rules" being both calming and humiliating or provoking, or locked doors giving rise to both protest and feelings of being cared for. Another important issue is the intersection of safety and dignity in psychiatric inpatient settings: for instance, the practice of removing potentially harmful items from patients upon admission has been indicated as having an impact on patient dignity, despite its importance for safety reasons, e.g. to prevent self-harm (Plunkett & Kelly, 2021; Plunkett et al., 2022).

Another study suggested that dignity within the psychiatric ward encompasses the preservation of self-identity and social roles, where patients feel a profound need to maintain their sense of self and societal connections despite the distress caused by severe mental illness. This involves the need of receiving acknowledgement and respect for their personal history, characteristics, and the continuation of social interactions to affirm their place in society (Di Lorenzo et al., 2017; Plunkett & Kelly, 2021). Additionally, managing emotional distress and uncertainty about the future is pivotal. These feelings often stem from the fear of losing control over one's life and worries about long-term outcomes, which are exacerbated by the hospital environment. Lastly, perceived autonomy was a fundamental dimension of dignity, challenged by restrictions of personal freedom and privacy (Di Lorenzo et al., 2017). Ensuring that these aspects are addressed in care practices is essential to upholding dignity in psychiatric settings (Plunkett & Kelly, 2021; Plunkett et al., 2022).

Professionals and caregivers also grapple with their roles as enforcers of coercive measures, and may be subject to "moral distress" and burnout (Jansen et al., 2020). Many healthcare providers experience deep ethical dilemmas, balancing the need for safety and clinical stability against respecting patient autonomy. The discomfort amongst professionals stems from the tension between clinical judgement and the coercive nature of some interventions deemed necessary for safety or treatment adherence (Aragonés-Calleja & Sánchez-Martínez, 2024; Wullschleger et al., 2024). The attitude is shifting from a therapeutic paradigm (coercive measures have positive effects on patients) to a safety paradigm (coercive measures are undesirable, but necessary for safety) (Doedens et al., 2020). Caregivers and relatives, whilst occasionally relieved that their loved ones are receiving care, express frustration and anxiety about the coercive processes. They often feel excluded from treatment decisions, which exacerbates their distress and complicates their relationships with both the patient and the healthcare system (Aragonés-Calleja & Sánchez-Martínez, 2024).

Coercion is an "elephant in the room": an understudied issue, despite its enormous relevance. There is a critical need for ongoing dialogue and ethical reflection in the application of coercion in mental health settings. There is also a strong need to implementing trauma-informed care practices within psychiatric facilities to better address and potentially mitigate these severe psychological impacts (Dutra et al., 2022). Effective management strategies suggested include staff training in trauma-awareness and the integration of specific therapeutic interventions that focus on trauma resolution and patient autonomy (Berry et al., 2013).

3.2.3   Mood and Morale During Inpatient Treatment for Psychosis

The experience of psychosis in itself and coercive treatment might constitute a "double hit" for the individual's sense of self-worth, mood, hope, morale. The dire consequences on individual morale depend on various individual and contextual factors, amongst which insight plays an important role. Enhanced insight into one's mental health is a desirable condition, but it can paradoxically lead to adverse outcomes, a phenomenon often referred to as the "insight paradox" (Belvederi Murri et al., 2015, 2016; Lysaker et al., 2007). This paradox suggests that insight can also lead to increased distress and depression. This is particularly evident in cases of post-psychotic depression, where patients who gain a clear awareness of their psychosis often experience a profound sense of loss and sadness over their perceived decline in personal and social identity. It is particularly evident amongst people who hold self-stigmatizing beliefs.

Demoralization may also manifest in patients with chronic psychotic illnesses, but also affective disorders, as loss of hope after a lifetime of struggling with an illness (Grassi et al., 2020) and may be expressed as reduced quality of life. The core lived experiences of the later stages of psychosis (i.e. relapsing and chronic) involved grieving personal losses, feeling split, and struggling to accept the constant inner chaos, the new self, the diagnosis, and an uncertain future (Fusar-Poli et al., 2022). Receiving treatment for chronic psychosis and having good insight into the illness also engender demoralization. This greater awareness of the illness, the realization of its the chronic course and the impact on personal and professional aspirations. As patients become more cognizant of how they are perceived and treated by others due to their illness, this can exacerbate feelings of hopelessness and low self-worth. However, this effect is tempered by better relationship with the carers (Belvederi Murri et al., 2016). The insight paradox encapsulates the dual-edged nature of awareness in psychiatric conditions.

On one hand, insight can empower patients, allowing for better self-management and informed decision-making; on the other, it can heighten awareness of stigma, the possible chronicity of their condition, and the impact on their life goals, thereby contributing to depressive symptoms or even suicide (Berardelli et al., 2021). Addressing the insight paradox in treatment planning involves a delicate balance. It requires fostering an environment that promotes insight whilst simultaneously providing robust emotional support and therapeutic interventions to mitigate the distressing impact of such insights. This nuanced understanding of insight and its implications is critical in psychiatric care, especially for ensuring that the pursuit of awareness does not inadvertently harm those it intends to help.

3.3   PSYCHOSIS AND EPISTEMIC (IN)JUSTICE

One last point should be made about the risk of epistemic injustice across the individual, social, or institutional scales (Kidd et al., 2023). The concept of epistemic injustice is particularly relevant both for the consequences of psychosis (as a clinical phenomenon) and for the experience of treatment. Epistemic injustice, in fact, concerns the lack of fairness in the exchange of knowledge, a domain that is particularly relevant to the experience of delusions. Individuals with psychosis often find themselves at the intersection of testimonial and hermeneutic injustices, where their capacity to know and communicate their experiences is unfairly discounted due to the nature of the illness and to the internal or external stigmatization of their condition (Kidd et al., 2022; Smyth, 2021).

Testimonial injustice relates to situations when an individual's account of their experiences is disregarded or deemed unreliable, not because of the content of their testimony, but because of prejudicial beliefs about their capacity to know ("identity-prejudicial" stereotype). For individuals with psychosis, this form of injustice is all too common, as the hallmark symptoms of their condition—delusions and hallucinations—are often dismissed as mere artefacts of their illness, rather than expressions of lived reality (Kidd et al., 2022; Smyth, 2021).

This may particularly interest patients with psychosis who are judged not to have capacity, and are considered completely unreliable in all aspects of their testimony, not just in regard to the content of a particular delusion or hallucination. This is obviously not true, as several degrees of detachment from reality exist in the psychotic spectrum, even in the acute phase (Smyth, 2021). Psychosis does not necessarily invade all realms of mental functioning and in many instances, patients may experience "lucid delusions" (not confused) and hold reliable accounts of a large proportion of their reality, events, experience. This is entrusted in the dialectic process of supporting decision-making in cases where capacity is lacking: the Mental Capacity Act requires practitioners to help a person make their own decision, before deciding that they are unable to make a decision (NICE Guidance, 2018).

The automatic dismissal of the testimony of people with psychosis silences their voices, and impedes their recovery by fostering feelings of isolation, alienation from the healthcare system and society at large, (Lysaker & Lysaker, 2010). Even in those cases where psychotic states may reduce the testimonial reliability of a person within a specific domain or a situation, the situation should be evaluated carefully depending on the observer's perspective, considering differences between laypeople, loved ones, and mental health professionals.

The closer one is to the person, the more one is invested by the task of attempting to understand and *interpret* psychosis as a different type of communication, both in the formal (Folesani et al., 2023) and substantial manner (Robbins, 2002; Stanghellini, 2008). In one interpretation, it could be argued that a person experiencing psychosis does also risk to commit testimonial injustice on themselves, by judging the self-experience of the world less reliable than it actually is, and by developing what is called self- or internalized stigma, which is particularly relevant for subsequent loss of self-esteem (Fernández et al., 2023).

Hermeneutic injustice is the other side of the coin of epistemic injustice in psychosis. The phenomenological tradition is particularly fit to capture the various, unique ways the embodied subject encounters the world, and how different it may be from their "neuro-normative" counterparts.

From other perspectives, the presence of cognitive impairment and other "dysfunctions", the difficulty of finding a shared language (Andreasen & Grove, 1986) and framework to articulate the complex and often ineffable nature of psychotic experiences may exacerbates patient marginalization, hindering effective communication with caregivers, healthcare providers, and the broader community (Heydebrand et al., 2004; Stanghellini et al., 2019; Tranulis et al., 2008). This form of injustice deprives individuals with psychosis of the opportunity to make sense of their experiences and to be understood by others, further isolating them and impeding their recovery.

There are several other relevant points that might pertain to epistemic injustice within the treatment of psychosis, but go beyond the scope of this chapter, such as stigma, objectification and misrecognition, hermeneutical marginalization and silencing (Kidd et al., 2017). It would be important to mention at least the analysis of institutional characteristics and rules that may exacerbate prejudice and miscommunication, including undue societal influences that influence the admission of patients. Specific attention should be devoted to the subjective worldview and experience of individuals with psychosis within the acute setting.

3.4   EVOLUTION OF PRINCIPLES OF CARE AND THE REDUCTION OF RESOURCES

More research is needed on the issues of dignity, demoralization, trauma, and epistemic injustice in the care for psychosis. At present, indications are on how to reduce hospitalizations altogether, or to reduce involuntary treatment. To a large extent, they depend on providing better care in the community. For instance, interventions may include patient-centred structured care planning with tools like crisis cards, advance directives, and continuous follow-up in the community; specialized therapeutic interventions such as animal-assisted psychotherapy, and acceptance and commitment therapy; and systemic changes in hospital practice comprising residential crisis programmes combining elements of residential and outpatient care (Giacco et al., 2018). Advance directives and crisis plans evidently constitute a strategy based on partnering with the patient and strengthening therapeutic alliance, a fundamental element for building trust and collaboration even in the most difficult clinical situations.

Other interventions can effectively reduce coercive treatments in mental health services. Amongst these, staff training showed the strongest evidence for reducing the use of restraints. Of note, this should not be limited to technical aspects, but also include relational and vocational aspects (Nesset et al., 2009). Targeted training and involving patients more actively in treatment decisions can help mitigate the use of coercive measures in mental health settings (Barbui et al., 2021). One interesting and innovative step is the direct involvement of persons who experience psychosis in psychiatry research. Patients bring unique insights (testimony) to the table to enhance the quality and effectiveness of inpatient psychiatric services. Employing participatory methods, new evaluative scales, and trials to test interventions can be further adapted to the needs of those who need them.

The last element to improve dignity of care is the resources of the mental healthcare system, another under-researched issue pertaining the correspondence between resources and quality of care (Barbui et al., 2018; Rickli et al., 2024). The paradox is that principles of care evolve, and we increasingly recognize the importance and role of humane and dignity-preserving care, but resources to put such principles into practice continue to wane, at least within the public mental healthcare sector. Any initiative to reduce compulsory treatments and coercion requires investment (Quinn et al., 2024). Italy, for instance, embodies this paradox by being a pioneer in the post-asylum change of paradigm for mental health, and being last amongst high-income countries for investment in public mental health, both in terms of monetary and human resources. Several countries may claim low overall rates of compulsory admissions, but too few data are available on the use of other formal and informal coercive measures (Bak & Aggernæs, 2012; Barbui et al., 2018; Starace, 2024). The levels of resources may be inversely proportional to the quantity of prescribed medications, lead to the hypothesis that increased personnel may allow for more non-pharmacological interventions, reducing the need for antipsychotics (Starace et al., 2018).

In conclusion, the experience of psychosis and its treatment in the emergency and inpatient setting often entails the dramatic necessity of compulsory treatment. These situations pose compelling ethical issues and endanger patient dignity, agency, and epistemic justice. Research on these issues is scarce, considering the dire consequences for individuals, but the available studies highlight several areas of improvement and hope for the possibility of humane treatment. It is paramount that the evolution of principles of care is accompanied by a parallel increase of resources to put such principles into practice.

Acknowledgements   Martino Belvederi Murri and Luigi Grassi acknowledge the support of project EPIC (Epistemic Injustice in Healthcare, 2023–2029), generously funded by a Wellcome Discovery Award and led by Havi Carel at the University of Bristol.

REFERENCES

Andreasen, N. C., & Grove, W. M. (1986). Thought, language, and communication in schizophrenia: Diagnosis and prognosis. *Schizophrenia Bulletin, 12*(3), 348–359. https://doi.org/10.1093/schbul/12.3.348

Aragonés-Calleja, M., & Sánchez-Martínez, V. (2024). Evidence synthesis on coercion in mental health: An umbrella review. *International Journal of Mental Health Nursing, 33*(2), 259–280. https://doi.org/10.1111/inm.13248

Badano, V. (2024). The Basaglia Law. Returning dignity to psychiatric patients: The historical, political and social factors that led to the closure of psychiatric hospitals in Italy in 1978. *History of Psychiatry* 957154X231224650. https://doi.org/10.1177/0957154X231224650

Bak, J., & Aggernæs, H. (2012). Coercion within Danish psychiatry compared with 10 other European countries. *Nordic Journal of Psychiatry, 66*(5), 297–302. https://doi.org/10.3109/08039488.2011.632645

Barbui, C., Purgato, M., Abdulmalik, J., Caldas-de-Almeida, J.M., Eaton, J., Gureje, O., Hanlon, C., Nosè, M., Ostuzzi, G., Saraceno, B., & Saxena, S. (2021). Efficacy of interventions to reduce coercive treatment in mental health services: Umbrella review of randomised evidence. *The British Journal of Psychiatry: The Journal of Mental Science, 218*(4), 185–195. https://doi.org/10.1192/bjp.2020.144

Barbui, C., Papola, D., & Saraceno, B. (2018). Forty years without mental hospitals in Italy. *International Journal of Mental Health Systems, 12*, 43. https://doi.org/10.1186/s13033-018-0223-1

Beaglehole, B., Beveridge, J., Campbell-Trotter, W., & Frampton, C. (2017). Unlocking an acute psychiatric ward: The impact on unauthorised absences, assaults and seclusions. *Bjpsych Bulletin, 41*(2), 92–96. https://doi.org/10.1192/pb.bp.115.052944

Belvederi Murri, M., Respino, M., Innamorati, M., Cervetti, A., Calcagno, P., Pompili, M., Lamis, D. A., Ghio, L., & Amore, M. (2015). Is good insight associated with depression among patients with schizophrenia? Systematic review and meta-analysis. *Schizophrenia Research, 162*(1–3), 234–247. https://doi.org/10.1016/j.schres.2015.01.003

Belvederi Murri, M., Amore, M., Calcagno, P., Respino, M., Marozzi, V., Masotti, M., Bugliani, M., Innamorati, M., Pompili, M., Galderisi, S., & Maj, M. (2016). The 'insight paradox' in schizophrenia: Magnitude, moderators and mediators of the association between insight and depression. *Schizophrenia Bulletin, 42*(5), 1225–1233. https://doi.org/10.1093/schbul/sbw040

Belvederi Murri, M., Zotos, S., Cantarelli, L., Berardi, L., Curtarello, E., Folesani, F., Gullotta, B., Bertolini, E., Girotto, B., Carozza, P., & Grassi, L. (2021a). Between China and Italy: A case report of first-episode schizophrenia in the Covid-19 era. *Psychiatry Research, 298*, 113804. https://doi.org/10.1016/j.psychres.2021.113804

Belvederi Murri, M., Bertelli, R., Carozza, P., Berardi, L., Cantarelli, L., Croce, E., Antenora, F., Curtarello, E. M. A., Simonelli, G., Recla, E., & Girotto, B. (2021b). First-episode psychosis in the Ferrara Mental Health Department: Incidence and clinical course within the first 2 years. *Early Intervention in Psychiatry, 15*(6), 1738–1748. https://doi.org/10.1111/eip.13095

Belvederi Murri, M., Ferrara, M., Imbesi, M., Leuci, E., Marchi, M., Musella, V., Natali, A., Neri, A., Ragni, S., Saponaro, A., & Tarricone, I. (2023). A public early intervention approach to first-episode psychosis: Treated incidence over 7 years in the Emilia-Romagna region. *Early Intervention in Psychiatry, 17*(7), 724–736. https://doi.org/10.1111/eip.13437

Belvederi Murri, M., & Amore, M. (2018). The multiple dimensions of insight in schizophrenia-spectrum disorders. *Schizophrenia Bulletin.* https://doi.org/10.1093/schbul/sby092

Berardelli, I., Innamorati, M., Sarubbi, S., Rogante, E., Erbuto, D., De Pisa, E., Costanza, A., Del Casale, A., Pasquini, M., Lester, D., & Pompili, M. (2021). Are demoralization and insight involved in suicide risk? An observational study on psychiatric inpatients. *Psychopathology, 54*(3), 127–135. https://doi.org/10.1159/000515056

Berry, K., Ford, S., Jellicoe-Jones, L., & Haddock, G. (2013). PTSD symptoms associated with the experiences of psychosis and hospitalisation: A review of the literature. *Clinical Psychology Review, 33*(4), 526–538. https://doi.org/10.1016/j.cpr.2013.01.011

Bø, B., Ottesen, Ø. H., Gjestad, R., Jørgensen, H. A., Kroken, R. A., Løberg, E. M., & Johnsen, E. (2016). Patient satisfaction after acute admission for psychosis. *Nordic Journal of Psychiatry, 70*(5), 321–328. https://doi.org/10.3109/08039488.2015.1112831

Burns, T., Rugkåsa, J., Yeeles, K., & Catty, J. (2016). *Coercion in mental health: A trial of the effectiveness of community treatment orders and an investigation of informal coercion in community mental health care.* Programme Grants for Applied Research. NIHR Journals Library.

Clement, S., Schauman, O., Graham, T., Maggioni, F., Evans-Lacko, S., Bezborodovs, N., Morgan, C., Rüsch, N., Brown, J. S., & Thornicroft, G. (2015). What is the impact of mental health-related stigma on help-seeking? A systematic review of quantitative and qualitative studies. *Psychological Medicine, 45*(1), 11–27. https://doi.org/10.1017/S0033291714000129

David, A. S. (1990). Insight and psychosis. *The British Journal of Psychiatry: The Journal of Mental Science, 156*, 798–808. https://doi.org/10.1192/bjp.156.6.798

David, A. S. (2020). Insight and psychosis: The next 30 years. *The British Journal of Psychiatry: The Journal of Mental Science, 217*(3), 521–523. https://doi.org/10.1192/bjp.2019.217

Di Lorenzo, R., Cabri, G., Carretti, E., Galli, G., Giambalvo, N., Rioli, G., Saraceni, S., Spiga, G., Del Giovane, C., & Ferri, P. (2017). A preliminary study of Patient Dignity Inventory validation among patients hospitalized in an acute psychiatric ward. *Neuropsychiatric Disease and Treatment, 13*, 177–190. https://doi.org/10.2147/NDT.S122423

Doedens, P., Vermeulen, J., Boyette, L.-L., Latour, C., & de Haan, L. (2020). Influence of nursing staff attitudes and characteristics on the use of coercive measures in acute mental health services—A systematic review. *Journal of Psychiatric and Mental Health Nursing, 27*(4), 446–459. https://doi.org/10.1111/jpm.12586

Douglas, L., Donohue, G., & Morrissey, J. (2022). Patient experience of physical restraint in the acute setting: A systematic review of the qualitative research evidence. *Issues in Mental Health Nursing, 43*(5), 473–481. https://doi.org/10.1080/01612840.2021.1978597

Dutra, P. E. P., Quagliato, L. A., & Nardi, A. E. (2022). Improving the perception of respect for and the dignity of inpatients: A systematic review. *British Medical Journal Open, 12*(5), e059129. https://doi.org/10.1136/bmjopen-2021-059129

Fernández, D., Grandón, P., López-Angulo, Y., Vladimir-Vielma, A., Peñate, W., & Díaz-Pérez, G. (2023). Internalized stigma and self-stigma in people diagnosed with a mental disorder. One concept or two? A scoping review. *The International Journal of Social Psychiatry, 69*(8), 1869–1881. https://doi.org/10.1177/00207640231196749

Folesani, F., Murri, M. B., Puggioni, C., Tiberto, E., Marella, M., Toffanin, T., Zerbinati, L., Nanni, M. G., Caruso, R., Brunato, D., & Ravelli, A. A. (2023). Linguistic markers of demoralization improvement in schizophrenia: A pilot study. *The European Journal of Psychiatry, 37*(3), 149–159. https://doi.org/10.1016/j.ejpsy.2023.03.001

Foucault, M., Murphy, J., & Khalfa, J. (2013). *History of madness*. Routledge.

Fusar-Poli, P., Estradé, A., Stanghellini, G., Venables, J., Onwumere, J., Messas, G., Gilardi, L., Nelson, B., Patel, V., Bonoldi, I., & Aragona, M. (2022).

The lived experience of psychosis: A bottom-up review co-written by experts by experience and academics. *World Psychiatry, 21*(2), 168–188. https://doi.org/10.1002/wps.20959

Giacco, D., Conneely, M., Masoud, T., Burn, E., & Priebe, S. (2018). Interventions for involuntary psychiatric inpatients: A systematic review. *European Psychiatry, 54*, 41–50. https://doi.org/10.1016/j.eurpsy.2018.07.005

Gooding, P., McSherry, B., & Roper, C. (2020). Preventing and reducing 'coercion' in mental health services: An international scoping review of English-language studies. *Acta Psychiatrica Scandinavica, 142*(1), 27–39. https://doi.org/10.1111/acps.13152

Grassi, L., Pasquini, M., Kissane, D., Zerbinati, L., Caruso, R., Sabato, S., Nanni, M. G., Ounalli, H., Maraone, A., Roselli, V., & Murri, M. B. (2020). Exploring and assessing demoralization in patients with non-psychotic affective disorders. *Journal of Affective Disorders, 274*, 568–575. https://doi.org/10.1016/j.jad.2020.05.043

Guzmán-Parra, J., Aguilera-Serrano, C., García-Sanchez, J. A., García-Spínola, E., Torres-Campos, D., Villagrán, J. M., Moreno-Küstner, B., & Mayoral-Cleries, F. (2019). Experience coercion, post-traumatic stress, and satisfaction with treatment associated with different coercive measures during psychiatric hospitalization. *International Journal of Mental Health Nursing, 28*(2), 448–456. https://doi.org/10.1111/inm.12546

Henriksen, M. G., & Parnas, J. (2014). Self-disorders and schizophrenia: A phenomenological reappraisal of poor insight and noncompliance. *Schizophrenia Bulletin, 40*(3), 542–547. https://doi.org/10.1093/schbul/sbt087

Heydebrand, G., Weiser, M., Rabinowitz, J., Hoff, A. L., DeLisi, L. E., & Csernansky, J. G. (2004). Correlates of cognitive deficits in first episode schizophrenia. *Schizophrenia Research, 68*, 1–9. https://doi.org/10.1016/S0920-9964(03)00097-5

Hoff, P. (2015). Medical-ethical guidelines: Coercive measures in medicine—Swiss Academy of Medical Sciences. *Swiss Medical Weekly.* https://doi.org/10.4414/smw.2015.14234

Huf, G., Coutinho, E. S. F., Adams, C. E., & Group, T.-S. C. (2012). Physical restraints versus seclusion room for management of people with acute aggression or agitation due to psychotic illness (TREC-SAVE): A randomized trial. *Psychological Medicine, 42*(11), 2265–2273. https://doi.org/10.1017/S0033291712000372

Isohanni, M., Nieminen, P., Moring, J., Pylkkänen, K., & Spalding, M. (1991). The dilemma of civil rights versus the right to treatment: Questionable involuntary admissions to a mental hospital. *Acta Psychiatrica Scandinavica, 83*(4), 256–261. https://doi.org/10.1111/j.1600-0447.1991.tb05536.x

Jansen, T.-L., Hem, M. H., Dambolt, L. J., & Hanssen, I. (2020). Moral distress in acute psychiatric nursing: Multifaceted dilemmas and demands. *Nursing Ethics, 27*(5), 1315–1326. https://doi.org/10.1177/0969733019877526

Jarrett, M., Bowers, L., & Simpson, A. (2008). Coerced medication in psychiatric inpatient care: Literature review. *Journal of Advanced Nursing, 64*(6), 538–548. https://doi.org/10.1111/j.1365-2648.2008.04832.x

Keane, S., Szigeti, A., Fanning, F., & Clarke, M. (2019). Are patterns of violence and aggression at presentation in patients with first-episode psychosis temporally stable? A comparison of 2 cohorts. *Early Intervention in Psychiatry, 13*(4), 888–894. https://doi.org/10.1111/eip.12694

Kidd, I. J., Medina, J., & Pohlhaus, G. (2017). The Routledge handbook of epistemic injustice.

Kidd, I. J., Spencer, L., & Carel, H. (2022). Epistemic injustice in psychiatric research and practice. *Philosophical Psychology*, 1–29. https://doi.org/10.1080/09515089.2022.2156333

Kidd, I. J., Spencer, L., & Harris, E. (2023). Epistemic injustice should matter to psychiatrists. *Philosophy of Medicine, 4*(1). https://doi.org/10.5195/pom.2023.159

Kirmayer, L. J., & Looper, K. J. (2006). Abnormal illness behaviour: Physiological, psychological and social dimensions of coping with distress. *Current Opinion in Psychiatry.* https://doi.org/10.1097/01.yco.0000194810.760 96.f2

Knight, S., Jarvis, G. E., Ryder, A. G., Lashley, M., & Rousseau, C. (2022). Ethnoracial differences in coercive referral and intervention among patients with first-episode psychosis. *Psychiatric Services (Washington, D.C.), 73*(1), 2–8. https://doi.org/10.1176/appi.ps.202000715

Kuipers, E., Yesufu-Udechuku, A., Taylor, C., & Kendall, T. (2014). Management of psychosis and schizophrenia in adults: Summary of updated NICE guidance. *BMJ, 348.*

Large, M. M., Nielssen, O., Ryan, C. J., & Hayes, R. (2008). Mental health laws that require dangerousness for involuntary admission may delay the initial treatment of schizophrenia. *Social Psychiatry and Psychiatric Epidemiology, 43*(3), 251–256. https://doi.org/10.1007/s00127-007-0287-8

Larkin, A., & Hutton, P. (2017). Systematic review and meta-analysis of factors that help or hinder treatment decision-making capacity in psychosis. *British Journal of Psychiatry, 211*(4), 205–215. https://doi.org/10.1192/bjp.bp.116.193458

Lorem, G. F., Hem, M. H., & Molewijk, B. (2015). Good coercion: Patients' moral evaluation of coercion in mental health care. *International Journal of Mental Health Nursing, 24*(3), 231–240. https://doi.org/10.1111/inm.12106

Lysaker, P. H., & Lysaker, J. T. (2010). Schizophrenia and alterations in self-experience: A comparison of 6 perspectives. *Schizophrenia Bulletin, 36*(2), 331–340. https://doi.org/10.1093/schbul/sbn077

Lysaker, P. H., Roe, D., & Yanos, P. T. (2007). Toward understanding the insight paradox: Internalized stigma moderates the association between insight and social functioning, hope, and self-esteem among people with schizophrenia spectrum disorders. *Schizophrenia Bulletin, 33*(1), 192–199. https://doi.org/10.1093/schbul/sbl016

Maiese, A., Dell'Aquila, M., Romano, S., Santurro, A., De Matteis, A., Scopetti, M., Arcangeli, M., & La Russa, R. (2019). Is it time for international guidelines on physical restraint in psychiatric patients? *La Clinica Terapeutica, 170*(1), e68–e70. https://doi.org/10.7417/CT.2019.2110

Maj, M., van Os, J., De Hert, M., Gaebel, W., Galderisi, S., Green, M. F., Guloksuz, S., Harvey, P. D., Jones, P. B., Malaspina, D., & McGorry, P. (2021). The clinical characterization of the patient with primary psychosis aimed at personalization of management. *World psychiatry: official journal of the World Psychiatric Association (WPA), 20*(1), 4–33. https://doi.org/10.1002/wps.20809

Nesset, M. B., Rossberg, J. I., Almvik, R., & Friis, S. (2009). Can a focused staff training programme improve the ward atmosphere and patient satisfaction in a forensic psychiatric hospital? A pilot study. *Scandinavian Journal of Caring Sciences, 23*(1), 117–124. https://doi.org/10.1111/j.1471-6712.2008.00597.x

NICE Guidance. (2018, October 3). *Recommendations on decision-making and mental capacity*. Available at https://www.nice.org.uk/guidance/ng108/chapter/recommendations. Last accessed 28 April 2024.

O'Brien, A. J., & Golding, C. G. (2003). Coercion in mental healthcare: The principle of least coercive care. *Journal of Psychiatric and Mental Health Nursing, 10*(2), 167–173. https://doi.org/10.1046/j.1365-2850.2003.00571.x

Plunkett, R., & Kelly, B. D. (2021). Dignity: The elephant in the room in psychiatric inpatient care? A systematic review and thematic synthesis. *International Journal of Law and Psychiatry, 75*, 101672. https://doi.org/10.1016/j.ijlp.2021.101672

Plunkett, R., O'Callaghan, A. K., & Kelly, B. D. (2022). Dignity, coercion and involuntary psychiatric care: A study of involuntary and voluntary psychiatry inpatients in Dublin. *International Journal of Psychiatry in Clinical Practice, 26*(3), 269–276. https://doi.org/10.1080/13651501.2021.2022162

Quinn, M., Jutkowitz, E., Primack, J., Lenger, K., Rudolph, J., Trikalinos, T., Rickard, T., Mai, H. J., Balk, E., & Konnyu, K. (2024). Protocols to reduce seclusion in inpatient mental health units. *International Journal of Mental Health Nursing*. https://doi.org/10.1111/inm.13277

Rickli, C., Stoll, J., Westermair, A. L., & Trachsel, M. (2024). Comparing attitudes towards compulsory interventions in severe and persistent mental illness among psychiatrists in India and Switzerland. *BMC Psychiatry, 24*(1), 295. https://doi.org/10.1186/s12888-024-05710-6

Robbins, M. (2002). The language of schizophrenia and the world of delusion. *The International Journal of Psychoanalysis, 83*(2), 383–405. https://doi.org/10.1516/ATTU-2M15-HX4F-5R2V

Sibitz, I., Scheutz, A., Lakeman, R., Schrank, B., Schaffer, M., & Amering, M. (2011). Impact of coercive measures on life stories: qualitative study. *The British Journal of Psychiatry, 199*(3), 239–244. https://doi.org/10.1192/bjp.bp.110.087841

Smyth, A. (2021). *Epistemic injustice in cases of compulsory psychiatric treatment.* University of Melbourne.

Stanghellini, G. (2008). Schizophrenic delusions, embodiment, and the background. *Philosophy, Psychiatry, & Psychology, 15*(4), 311–314.

Stanghellini, G., Broome, M., Raballo, A., Fernandez, A. V., Fusar-Poli, P., & Rosfort, R. (2019). *The Oxford handbook of phenomenological psychopathology.* Oxford University Press.

Starace, F. (2024). *Rapporto SIEP 2024. La salute mentale nell'Italia del regionalismo.* Youcanprint.

Starace, F., Mungai, F., & Barbui, C. (2018). Does mental health staffing level affect antipsychotic prescribing? Analysis of Italian national statistics. *PLoS ONE, 13*(2), e0193216. https://doi.org/10.1371/journal.pone.0193216

Stovell, D., Wearden, A., Morrison, A. P., & Hutton, P. (2016). Service users' experiences of the treatment decision-making process in psychosis: A phenomenological analysis. *Psychosis, 8*(4), 311–323. https://doi.org/10.1080/17522439.2016.1145730

Tranulis, C., Corin, E., & Kirmayer, L. J. (2008). Insight and psychosis: Comparing the perspectives of patient, entourage and clinician. *The International Journal of Social Psychiatry, 54*(3), 225–241. https://doi.org/10.1177/0020764008088860

Valenti, E., Banks, C., Calcedo-Barba, A., Bensimon, C. M., Hoffmann, K. M., Pelto-Piri, V., Jurin, T., Mendoza, O. M., Mundt, A. P., Rugkåsa, J., & Tubini, J. (2015). Informal coercion in psychiatry: A focus group study of attitudes and experiences of mental health professionals in ten countries. *Social Psychiatry and Psychiatric Epidemiology, 50*(8), 1297–1308. https://doi.org/10.1007/s00127-015-1032-3

Walsh, E., Buchanan, A., & Fahy, T. (2002). Violence and schizophrenia: Examining the evidence. *The British Journal of Psychiatry, 180*(6), 490–495. https://doi.org/10.1192/bjp.180.6.490

Witt, K., van Dorn, R., & Fazel, S. (2013). Risk factors for violence in psychosis: Systematic review and meta-regression analysis of 110 studies. *PLoS ONE, 8*(2), e55542. https://doi.org/10.1371/journal.pone.0055942

Wullschleger, A., Chatton, A., Kuenzi, N., Baeriswyl, R., Kaiser, S., & Bartolomei, J. (2024). Experience of violence and attitudes of staff members towards coercion in psychiatric settings: Observational study. *BJPsych Open*, *10*(3), e80. https://doi.org/10.1192/bjo.2024.29

Zaami, S., Rinaldi, R., Bersani, G., & Marinelli, E. (2020). Restraints and seclusion in psychiatry: striking a balance between protection and coercion. Critical overview of international regulations and rulings. *Rivista Di Psichiatria*, *55*(1), 16–23. https://doi.org/10.1708/3301.32714

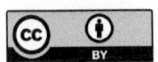

Not All Psychiatric Diagnoses are Created Equal: Comparing Depression and Borderline Personality Disorders

Jay Watts

Abstract The validity of psychiatric diagnoses has been at the heart of enduring and divisive debates in mental health discourse for over fifty years, often reaching a stalemate. Whilst some consider a diagnosis essential for validation and support, others view it as an obstacle to personal meaning-making. This chapter proposes that considering epistemic injustice may offer a valuable approach to overcome this impasse. By examining four facets of epistemic injustice—objectification, moral agency, trivialization, and narrative agency—it juxtaposes patient perspectives on borderline personality disorder and depression, arguably the least and most popular diagnoses with patients in psychiatry. Leveraging these four facets, it delves into the experiences of two representative patients, Cara and John, showing how epistemic injustice operates differently across diagnoses. This analysis suggests the importance of epistemic injustice as a tool in critically evaluating the usefulness of specific psychiatric diagnoses, enriching traditional metrics of reliability and validity in

J. Watts (✉)
Centre for Mental Health Research, City, University of London, London, UK
e-mail: clinic@jaywatts.co.uk

L. Bortolotti (ed.), *Epistemic Justice in Mental Healthcare*,
https://doi.org/10.1007/978-3-031-68881-2_4

nosology. Moreover, it encourages a shift in clinical training to embrace reflective practices and restructure power dynamics in clinical encounters, promoting greater epistemic participation.

Keywords Psychiatric diagnoses · Epistemic injustice · Testimonial injustice · Narrative agency · Diagnosis: psychiatric diagnosis · Mental health · Borderline personality disorder · Depression · Societal attitudes · Peer-led training

4.1   Are Psychiatric Diagnoses Meaningful?

Throughout the last half-century's societal tumult, the perception of psychiatric diagnosis has fluctuated, alternately emerging from, and receding into the shadows of cultural awareness. Previously, it lingered on the fringes, gaining attention primarily through countercultural critiques like Michel Foucault's 'Madness and Civilization' and R. D. Laing's ground-breaking work at Kingsley Hall. Now, however, these once-peripheral views have vaulted into the mainstream, taking a central place in public discourse. This transition mirrors a shift in societal attitudes towards mental illness. It has been accelerated by powerful stigma-reducing initiatives such as 'Time to Change' (Henderson & Thornicroft, 2009), as well as culturally defining moments that have shaped public emotion—notably, Paul 'Gazza' Gascoigne's poignant tears during the 1990 World Cup and the collective mourning following Princess Diana's death (Dixon, 2023).

Today, mental health discussions have moved from the seclusion of private spaces to dominate conversations everywhere—from boundless digital realms to the intimacy of family gatherings. Yet this newfound openness has its critics, warning of the medicalization of everyday life, casting doubt on the veracity of severe conditions like schizophrenia and claiming that young people especially are overidentifying with mental illness labels thanks to TikTok culture (e.g. Giedinghagen, 2023). Such polarized views—often referred to as 'the diagnosis wars'—are heated and sometimes unpleasant, frequently invalidating the experiences of those of us who have been diagnosed. Our experiences are nearly always more complex. For instance, my own feelings about my diagnoses vary; some feel affirming, others condemning.

Epistemic justice has emerged as a potent framework for conveying the complexities long articulated in Mad Writings (e.g. Russo & Sweeney, 2016). By exploring how epistemic injustice manifests in the context of two diagnoses—depression and borderline personality disorder (BPD)—I aim to show the epistemic traps that diagnosis can lead us into or help us escape from. Critically examining the ethics of psychiatric diagnoses becomes meaningful only if there is a substantial factual basis to question the diagnoses themselves, sufficient to warrant disagreement.

Psychiatric diagnostics aim to balance the need to categorize mental health conditions with the complexity of human experience. Diagnoses function as clusters of symptoms, assumed to coalesce as 'syndromes' which are given names such as 'depression' and 'schizophrenia,' purporting to provide insights into cause, course, treatment, and outcome. These classifications are judged on two key factors: *reliability*, or how consistent a diagnostic measure is, and *validity*, or how accurately the measure reflects what it's supposed to. Reliability and validity vary significantly between and within diagnoses. For example, Bipolar Affective Disorder has good construct validity, especially for Bipolar I, its most acute form, compared to Bipolar II (Cano-Ruiz et al., 2020).

In contrast to other medical disciplines that often rely on a blend of subjective symptoms and objective signs such as rashes or fevers, psychiatric diagnoses are primarily based on subjective observations, including reported mood and behavioural changes. The complexity of diagnosis is highlighted by the remarkable number of possible symptom combinations—for instance, there are 227 for major depressive disorder (Zimmerman et al., 2015) and 256 for borderline personality disorder (Hawkins et al., 2014).

Relying on subjective symptoms gives psychiatric diagnoses a value-laden and bias-prone quality that can delegitimize their status. However, Carl Sagan's axiom, "Absence of Evidence is not Evidence of Absence," resonates here. Whilst we might ridicule psychiatry's eternal expectation that biomarkers linked to syndromes are on the brink of being discovered, similar sign-less conditions in other medical areas, such as certain types of headaches, do not face the same degree of scepticism. Psychiatric diagnoses serve multiple purposes, including ruling out other medical conditions. For example, symptoms of depression can overlap with those of heart or thyroid problems, necessitating thorough diagnostic processes to discern and eliminate these alternatives.

Threshold points are debated across medicine. For example, the cut-off points for diabetes have changed over time. In psychiatry, they are especially problematic because deciding when sadness becomes depression or when eating problems become a disorder is a value-laden decision, influenced by time and place.

Mainstream critiques of psychiatric diagnosis often repeat many of the very issues they seek to contest such as over-generalizing claims or creating straw man arguments that misrepresent the biopsychosocial model as a biomedical one. There are also plenty of criticisms of the current syndrome-based diagnostic system from within mainstream psychiatry. For example, 2014's Research Domain Criteria (Insel, 2014) was led by NIMH's most prominent biomarker researchers. They advocate for symptom-level research, recognizing the transdiagnostic nature of most symptoms. Nassir Ghaemi, an influential supporter of RDoC, emphasizes the need for challenging the field: "It's uncomfortable for a lot of people, but the field needs to be pushed—hard" (Ledford, 2013).

Given these challenges and the complexity of psychiatric diagnoses, we must focus on two essential steps. First, we should avoid generalizing diagnoses as if they are uniform, recognizing the substantial variation in their reliability and validity. Second, we should emphasize another criterion: usefulness. To assess the usefulness of diagnoses, it is crucial to include the perspective of the often overlooked 'missing person' in the diagnostic process—the patient (Phillips, 2010).

According to Perkins and colleagues' excellent systematic review of this under-researched area, the impact of a diagnosis depends on its manner of delivery, patient interpretation, and its functional utility—specifically, whether it helps validate suffering and facilitates access to treatment (Perkins et al., 2018). A diagnosis that is effectively communicated can illuminate and empower, aiding patients in understanding and managing their conditions. In contrast, a diagnosis perceived as misaligned or impersonally delivered can exacerbate feelings of alienation and despair. Diagnoses do not perform equally on these fronts, with depression amongst the most positively received and personality disorders the least. This discrepancy should not be simplistically attributed to illness severity; Lived Experience Narratives suggest that a more fundamental issue is at play: a different level of prejudice affecting patients' capacity to be taken seriously as experts on their own experience (e.g. 'Recovery in the Bin, 2019'). Epistemic injustice may be a useful conceptual tool to understand and address these diagnostic disparities.

4.2   Epistemic Injustice in Psychiatry

Miranda Fricker's seminal work has introduced the concept of epistemic injustice (Fricker, 2007). In contrast to other forms of injustice, which may involve unequal distribution of physical resources such as food and shelter, epistemic injustice concerns problems in the distribution of belief, credibility, and meaning. This bifurcates into two main areas: testimonial and hermeneutical injustice. Testimonial injustice occurs "when prejudice causes a hearer to give a deflated level of credibility to a speaker's word;" hermeneutical injustice occurs "at a prior stage, when a gap in collective interpretive resources puts someone at an unfair disadvantage when it comes to making sense of their social experiences" (Fricker, 2007). If one party has a 'credibility excess,' identity prejudice may give undue weight to their contributions in an encounter. Conversely, another party may suffer from a 'credibility deficit' due to the identities they hold. Clinicians tend to have relative credibility excess in the psychiatric encounter, though this varies depending on profession, seniority, age, and so on.

The power dynamics in conversations are fluid, much like the coordinated movements of dancers. Through these interactions, speakers may experience shifts in credibility influenced by factors such as testimonial inflation and deflation, causing their credibility to either increase or decrease from moment to moment. These shifts extend beyond epistemic credibility and the explicit content of the conversation. Non-verbal cues, like eye contact, gestures, and the rhythm of speech, play a pivotal role. They involve how speech is integrated into the dialogue, such as how hesitations are treated—whether acknowledged respectfully or overlooked. Each of these elements adds a layer to the intricate dance of conversation (e.g. Schore, 2003).

When there is an extreme power imbalance or if a negative pattern has repeated often enough in a person's life, two additional forms of testimonial injustice, as identified by Kristie Dotson (2011), may emerge. Testimonial smothering occurs when individuals feel compelled to self-censor because their audience may not be receptive or supportive of their viewpoint. Testimonial quieting, on the other hand, involves the unfair diminishing of a speaker's credibility, often due to biases like racism, sexism, or other prejudices, which leads to their contributions being undervalued or ignored. These recurring patterns not only impact what Houlders and colleagues (2021) identify as 'epistemic agency'—a person's ability to competently and authoritatively produce and share knowledge—but also mould our very sense of self.

Our self-perception is often shaped by a subtle, internalized chorus of judgements. This phenomenon is vividly apparent in experiences like voice-hearing and is mirrored in theatrical traditions such as the Greek chorus. Our sense of self is relational; we absorb and replay interactions with others, particularly from early life, within our psyche's internal drama (Chen et al., 2006). These internalized interactions shape our engagement with the world and lead us to expect treatment echoing our past roles. Our 'narrative self' navigates the world using an autobiographical narrative that is not rigid but loosely structured, providing us continuity through time—past and future (Wortham, 2000). Selfhood is seen as a construct, constantly being rewritten and reshaped, both in response to present experiences and past events. Memory, here, is more malleable and subject to the hues of our current mood than we like to think (Schore, 2003).

Epistemic justice has become an increasingly recognized framework for understanding the complex power dynamics at play in psychiatry, both generally (e.g. Crichton et al., 2017; Kidd et al., 2023; Scrutton, 2017) and in relation to specific diagnoses (e.g. Borderline Personality Disorder—Watts, 2017; Depression—Jackson, 2017; OCD—Spencer & Carel, 2021). In this analysis, I will apply four themes derived from this literature—objectification (Sakakibara, 2023), moral agency (Houlders et al., 2021; Kyratsous & Sanati, 2017), trivialization (Spencer & Carel, 2021), and narrative agency (Bertilsdotter Rosqvist et al., 2023)—to illustrate the challenges faced by patients diagnosed with depression and BPD. *Objectification* occurs when patients are seen more as subjects of their diagnosis rather than as individuals. *Moral agency* pertains to the capacity of patients to make ethical decisions and be responsible for their actions. Depathologization seeks to reframe mental health conditions, not as pathological disorders, but as responses to life experiences or socio-cultural factors. However, this can lead to *trivialization*, where the severity or significance of a mental health condition is minimized or dismissed. *Narrative agency* is the person's ability to construct their experiences into a coherent story, shaping their own narrative. In psychiatric settings, this ability is often challenged, as patient narratives may not align with societal or clinical expectations.

Utilizing these four factors as our guide, let's shift our focus to the clinic and investigate how they may function when dealing with depression, one of the most practically beneficial diagnoses, and BPD, which is perhaps the least so.

4.3   Two Vignettes

4.3.1   John

John, a 32-year-old civil servant, sat numbly across from his GP, his mind as blank as the whitewashed walls of the office. His anguish wasn't just a recent affliction; it had roots stretching back to his youth, back to the days when John's father's stern gaze and biting words had etched a deep sense of inadequacy into his soul and into his sense of manhood and personhood.

'Depression' was the diagnosis the GP had given John, a word that echoed in his thoughts. It clashed violently with the image John held of himself—a man who should be strong, in control, unyielding to emotional tides. Depression was about feeling sad, wasn't it? John didn't weep or wail; he just felt… empty, a shell moving through life's motions.

John's girlfriend's laughter, which once filled him with such joy, now sounded like a foreign language. "It's nothing to be ashamed of, we all get sad sometimes," she'd said, her words unintentionally diminishing the gravity of his internal drought. If she got as sad as him, how could she get up to go to the gym and laugh with her mates? How come he was the one being accused of being 'disconnected'—well until she'd seen that advert from MIND about men's mental health, that is.

Amidst these struggles, John's best mate had offered his own brand of advice: "You just need a good night out with the boys," he'd joked, a comment that stung John more than it soothed. Yet, in this small, sterile room, with the GP's words floating in the air, something within John shifted. The idea that this relentless void within him had a name, that it wasn't merely a personal failing or lack of willpower, that it was an illness, was both terrifying and liberating. It was as if a faint light had flickered in the distance, a beacon suggesting a path out of the fog. Maybe he wasn't fundamentally flawed. Maybe he could dial the counselling service number his doctor had given to him. Maybe, just maybe, there was hope.

4.3.2   Cara

Cara's fingers trembled as she dialled the crisis line, her heart pounding with a mix of dread and faint hope. Her past—the yelling, the hurtful words, the feeling of being unwanted and unloved—washed over her like waves. She clutched the phone tighter, a lifeline in a sea of turmoil. As she waited for a response, flashes of her past overwhelmed her, making her heart race. When Sammi, the crisis worker, answered, his voice held a note of strained patience, as if he was bracing for yet another routine call.

Cara tried to speak, her words stumbling out in a rush. "I just... I saw this scene on TV, and it's like it's happening to me, all over again," her voice cracked, the rawness of her emotions laid bare.

Through the phone, she sensed Sammi's disinterest, his responses mechanical and distant. Each word from him felt like a dismissal, reinforcing her deepest fears—that she was just a case number, her pain merely another item on someone's checklist.

"It's not just a bad day, it's like I'm living in that moment again... with my stepdad," Cara stammered.

Sammi interrupted with a clinical tone. "Have you tried using your DBT skills, Cara? Maybe a bath to distract yourself?"

Cara's voice rose, tinged with frustration and desperation. "It's not about skills or baths! It's about feeling heard... safe."

There was a pause on the line, then Sammi's voice returned, flat and procedural. "Cara, are you having thoughts of harming yourself right now?"

The question, blunt and devoid of empathy, stung her. Cara wanted to scream, to make him understand, but instead, her voice broke. "I don't... I don't know." And then with more force, "I've got some pills and I..."

Sammi's reply was swift, almost dismissive. "Well, you wouldn't be calling us if you really wanted to kill yourself, now, would you?"

Cara's journey through the foster care system, which began at age 14, had been a labyrinth of misunderstandings and dismissals. She had been shuffled from one home to another, each move chipping away at her sense of self-worth. Cara's stepdad's manipulations to hide what he called 'their secret' had woven a narrative of her being 'dramatic,' 'attention-seeking,' and 'a problem child.' This label stuck, colouring every interaction, even with her mum who chose the path of denial over facing the painful truth.

The dial tone echoed in Cara's ears long after the call had ended. A mixture of rage and despair swirled within her. "I'll show them," she thought bitterly. She'd overdose then they'd get in trouble! But then Cara's anger quickly turned inward. "Perhaps they are right, I am manipulative," the familiar, scathing narrative whispered in her mind, reinforcing the hurtful labels she'd fought against, making the pills inviting in a different way.

4.4   COMPARATIVE ANALYSIS

At first glance, John and Cara's experiences may seem like examples of good versus poor care. However, Cara's experiences are far more routine than we might hope (Beale, 2022; Langley & Price, 2022) and are reflective of what the literature tells us patients are more likely to receive due to their diagnosis (Lomani et al., 2022; Recovery in the Bin, 2019). To understand why, it's worth familiarizing ourselves with some facts about depression and BPD.

Depression is a mental health disorder characterized by persistent sadness, loss of interest, and symptoms like sleep issues and fatigue (World Health Organization, 2022). Its severity can range from mild to severe. Often called the 'common cold' of mental illness, depression's widespread impact is sometimes misinterpreted, leading to stereotypical images. One such stereotype is the depiction of depression as a sad, crying woman, which, whilst aligning with the higher diagnosis rate in women, can discourage men from seeking help and contribute to a gender gap in suicide rates (Oliffe et al., 2019). In recent years, several successful anti-stigma campaigns have focused on depression, often under the banner of situating mental health as 'just like any other illness' (Henderson & Thornicroft, 2009). Treatments have been rolled out to a wider range of the public. The British Psychological Society's (2020) recent report on 'Understanding Depression,' misjudged the public mood, stirring controversy by highlighting the psychological and socio-cultural dimensions of depression and describing it as 'a common human experience.' This perspective drew a backlash for appearing to minimize the severity of the condition, as highlighted by one individual's response: 'I've been in intensive care and sectioned... But according to this report, I'm not ill... just experiencing something common" (Lucy's Depression Diary, 2020). Depression has relatively good construct validity for a psychiatric diagnosis (World Health Organization, 2022). The same cannot be said for BPD.

BPD is conceptualized as a mental health condition characterized by mood instability, impulsive behaviour, and challenging interpersonal relationships. As one of the most debated diagnoses in psychiatry, BPD is notorious for its high heterogeneity and levels of comorbidity (Hawkins et al., 2014), leading to it being seen as a 'dustbin diagnosis.' (Lomani et al., 2022) This label is often used for patients who do not fit neatly into traditional diagnostic categories or who may be unfavourably viewed by clinicians (e.g. Lomani et al., 2022). Patients with BPD are often perceived by healthcare professionals to be 'attention-seeking,' 'manipulative,' and 'overemotional' (e.g. Baker & Beazley, 2022) a view that can colour clinical interactions and potentially influence treatment outcomes (Lam et al., 2016).

Three out of four patients diagnosed with BPD are women, and 70% of all patients have experienced complex trauma, including sexual, emotional, and physical abuse (Vermetten & Spiegel, 2014). For many patients, being labelled with BPD is retraumatizing, no more than a 'sophisticated insult' that adds 'insult to injury' (Lomani et al., 2022). In response to these concerns, Complex Post-Traumatic Stress Disorder (CPTSD) was proposed as a more appropriate diagnosis to provide a more affirmative and less stigmatizing label for individuals predominantly affected by trauma (Herman, 2015). However, CPTSD, newly minted in the latest diagnostic manual, has stringent inclusion criteria that excludes as many trauma survivors as it includes (Watts, 2019). It is increasingly recognized that BPD's broad diagnostic criteria masks multiple underlying conditions, including undiagnosed autism (Watts, 2023a), contraindicating a one-size-fits-all solution.

BPD has been on the brink of removal from psychiatric nosology since its introduction in 1980 and was scheduled to be removed from the latest recent iteration of ICD until a last-minute U-turn fuelled by political lobbying (Mulder & Tyrer, 2023). Currently, it is awkwardly retained as a 'trait qualifier' in the new system categorizing personality disorders as mild, moderate, and severe. This retention, however, statistically collapses the new model, effectively satisfying no one (Watts, 2019). A 2018 Personality Disorder Consensus Statement by leading UK patient and professional organizations recognized some diversity in opinion about the label amongst patients but called for its removal given the potential iatrogenic harm (Lamb et al., 2018). Unlike 'Understanding Depression,' the Personality Disorder Consensus statement received little backlash.

The framing of BPD and depression profoundly influences the clinical encounters of individuals like John, Cara, and Sammi. By exploring four facets of epistemic injustice, we can better conceptualize the various obstacles they face.

4.4.1   Objectification

John's agony has not been recognized as depression because of a highly gendered stereotype of what it looks like—sadness, crying—that he, his girlfriend, and best mate share. John's emptiness and alienation have gone unregistered, his internal dramaturgy replicating his dad's 'biting words' against him, calling him weak and lacking in willpower. The medical diagnosis of John's condition provides a new lens, helping him to disengage his suffering from personal shortcomings. If he accepts counselling, his sense of agency may well increase. Therapy for depression is expansive, as it unpicks and narratively thickens the underlying issues, encouraging subjectification by allowing him to become an active participant in his own story.

Cara faces stark objectification, often being treated as 'a borderline' rather than as a person. Influenced by limited training and a pervasive 'backstage borderline talk' culture (Watts, 2023b), healthcare providers like Sammi tend to perceive individuals with BPD as 'manipulative' or 'attention-seeking.' This perpetuates a stigma, neither acknowledging them as truly unwell nor fully mentally ill. Misogynistic biases further fuel these views, depicting women with BPD as 'inconsistent' and 'over-dramatic.' Whilst Sammi's approach may have once been more empathic, he is likely to have been encouraged to adopt a more distant, managerial style for fear that Cara is 'splitting' the team. Such notions create a 'PD shield' that impedes genuine connection, reinforcing in Cara a sense that her emotions are excessive and unbearable (Watts, 2023b). The treatment alluded to, Dialectical Behaviour Therapy (DBT), is useful for some, but is constrictive rather than expansive, as treatment goals, such as reducing hospitalization days and self-harm, are predetermined by the state rather than tailored to her individual needs (Linehan, 1993).

The notion of BPD patients as having an 'unstable sense-of-self' exacerbates power imbalances in the clinician–patient relationship. Assumptions about Cara's fluctuating moods devalue her current feelings and thoughts. This overlooks the commonality of self-state shifts, especially in those who have experienced trauma or are neurodivergent (Watts, 2023b). Careful processing of trauma may allow for the differentiation between 'past' and 'present' experiences, and subsequently to fewer extreme reactions (e.g. Herman, 2015). Testimonial deflation hinders Cara from processing and integrating her trauma, leading to an increased likelihood of dissociation, consolidating the idea of her as unstable rather than desperate.

4.4.2   Moral Agency

John's depression, when understood medically, is detached from moral judgement. This framing positions his condition as an illness rather than a personal failing. Consequently, he is not perceived as morally culpable for his symptoms. Medicalization allows him to shift his perspective from viewing his issues as inherent flaws to recognizing them as challenges he faces. In contrast, Cara's experience with BPD is laden with moral judgement, as her challenges are perceived as inherent to her personality rather than as symptoms of a condition. This is especially problematic given that 85% of BPD patients experience recovery over a ten-year period with even the ICD Chair stating problems have little if anything to do with personality (Mulder & Tyrer, 2023). Ascription to personality places Cara in a troubling double bind: she is perceived as both childlike, lacking understanding of her needs due to her shifting self-states, and overly responsible for the outcomes of her actions. This dichotomy propels Cara into a 'witch's dilemma' regarding her suicidal intentions, where her sincerity is only likely to be accepted if she dies, despite the commonality of ambivalence in suicidal ideation.

Such paradoxes lead to dramatic fluctuations in Cara's emotional state, swinging from hyperadrenalization, where she strives to be heard energetically, to hypoarousal, marked by stuttering and resignation. Cara's 'mental capacity'—whether she is mentally capable of making decisions in her best interests—is presumed, though her suicidal ideation is not properly assessed. This presumption of capacity in BPD is notoriously dangerous, with suicide attempts written off as 'impulsive' and patients often receiving poor care in emergency rooms and crisis teams (Beale, 2022).

4.4.3   Trivialization

In John's case, societal responses to his depression, such as his friend's suggestion, "You just need a good night out with the boys," and his girlfriend's comment, "We all get sad sometimes," reflect a tendency to trivialize mental health issues. These interactions, aiming to normalize his symptoms, risk undermining the seriousness of his condition.

Cara's experience with BPD presents a contrasting dynamic. In clinical settings, her intense emotional displays and complex trauma responses are often seen as 'too much' for social acceptance, yet paradoxically, they are deemed 'too little' to warrant serious medical intervention. Comments from healthcare professionals that downplay her suicidality not only treat her emotional experiences as performative and functional but also feed into this cycle of trivialization. This perpetuates the narrative of her being simultaneously overwhelming in her needs yet not sufficiently ill to necessitate earnest medical attention, a cruel juxtaposition shaped by both born the enforced secrecy of her stepdad's abuse and society's inability to adequately categorize her pain.

4.4.4 Narrative Agency

The diagnosis of depression serves as a catalyst for John, enabling him to reconstruct his self-narrative. This framework allows him to cultivate relationships with himself that are nurturing and empathetic, a stark contrast to the internalized harshness and criticism inherited from his father's presence. This shift is significant as depression often embeds deep-seated beliefs of worthlessness and failure within an individual's psyche (Beck & Alford, 2009). As his diagnosis is a powerful, epistemically bolstered tool given to him by someone with relative epistemic credibility—a doctor— we might expect it to be picked up by his girlfriend, who might use it to rescue John from defeatist feelings about not waking up gym ready until, we hope, John is better.

Cara's narrative agency is drastically constrained by the objectification she experiences. Her attempts to mobilize what has been triggered by the TV program are repeatedly shut down, which is damaging because trauma can demand to be placed in autobiographical narrative so it can be time-stamped as past, enabling body and mind to feel safer in the present (Herman, 2015). The testimonial smothering and quieting not only remove that possibility from Cara but also limit treatment possibilities as she is placed in a diagnostic group where 'not all' patients have experienced trauma, meaning that it is decentred in practice (e.g. Linehan, 1993). This leaves Cara trapped in a discourse that reinforces a problem-saturated narrative (White & Epston, 1990) first introduced by her stepdad to ensure that his abuse of her was silenced. The repetition of the idea of her as 'attention-seeking' and 'manipulative' reinforces his script that she is the 'problem child' such that even though she tries to produce different relationships, she too comes to see herself as potentially at fault ("'Perhaps they are right, I am manipulative").

The issue here is deeply rooted in a misunderstanding of how powerful ideology and language are in shaping one's reality. In Cara's case, since the language surrounding her shapes her sense of self-worth, how can she see herself as deserving? This cycle rewrites her past and shapes her future, stripping her of the power to articulate her own story and leaving her struggling for words. She is trapped in a loop, influencing her identity and life choices.

The analysis of John and Cara's vignettes highlights significant differences in how mental health conditions are perceived and treated. Both are subject to hermeneutic injustice in that both are given relatively simple ideas of what is wrong—but the functional effects of this are very different. Whilst John's experience with depression allows for some degree of narrative control, acknowledgement, and absence of moral judgement, Cara's experience with BPD is riddled with objectification, moral judgement, trivialization, and constraints on her narrative agency. No diagnosis should shape the extent to which a person's rights are honoured or diminished.

4.5   Towards a More Equitable Psychiatric Practice

John and Cara's experiences demonstrate the epistemic possibilities and obstacles that different diagnoses can produce. Are these experiences universal? Of course not. However, they reflect common enough patterns associated with specific diagnoses to serve as a launching pad for broader thinking about the diagnostic system and the questions we might ask of our diagnoses.

Diagnoses are not merely clinical labels; they are complex constructs imbued with biases, stereotypes, and preconceived notions. These elements subtly influence both patients and providers, impacting patients' roles as knowers or contributors of knowledge. John and Cara's experiences highlight how psychiatric labels can lead to testimonial deflation or contribute to hermeneutic injustice, hindering meaningful engagement with patients' experiences. Whilst diagnoses can facilitate the articulation and recognition of pain, they can also dangerously delegitimize pain and perceived worthiness.

Decoupling diagnostic concepts from discourses that perpetuate prejudice is essential. This shift legitimizes patients' abilities to articulate their suffering and its origins and challenges the foundations on which psychiatric nosology is judged. Concerns about reliability and validity in psychiatry should not be seen merely as shortcomings but as opportunities to emphasize a third criterion—diagnoses' utility. Epistemic justice is a core component of this usefulness.

Through a more equitable psychiatric practice, we can better address not only specific cases, such as those of Cara and John, but also engage with broader questions of existing and potential diagnoses, including:

- **Objectification**: Does the diagnosis respect patient individuality, or does it contribute to stereotyping and dehumanization? How might it reinforce or challenge societal stereotypes?
- **Moral Agency**: How does this diagnosis affect perceptions of a patient's responsibility for their condition? Does it empower them in their treatment and recovery decisions?
- **Trivialization:** Does the diagnosis recognize and validate the seriousness of the patient's symptoms and experiences? Is there a risk of their concerns being dismissed, especially by healthcare professionals?
- **Narrative Agency**: Does this diagnosis enable or restrict a patient's ability to shape and express their own life story? How does it influence their ability to communicate individual experiences?

These questions must be considered within the broader context of historical biases and entrenched prejudices that shape our perceptions. The association of BPD with notions of hysteria and the weight of misogynistic prejudice makes it doubly unacceptable as a diagnosis due to its lack of reliability and validity, and the hefty weight of prejudice. These factors have led to scandalous treatment in psychiatry and frequently appear in public health scandals (e.g. Cumberlege, 2020). Despite decades of efforts to destigmatize BPD, these ingrained prejudices have made it nearly impossible (National Institute for Mental Health, 2003). Suggesting that someone can simply choose not to use a diagnosis is not viable and violates what we might call 'diagnostic rights,' including access to social support and treatment. Affirmative diagnostic alternatives must, therefore, be available (Watts, 2019).

Epistemic transformation can only occur within a wider tapestry that encourages an ethic of listening.

Steps to Foster Epistemic Collaboration:

- **Co-authorship and Patient Advocacy:** Involve patients in developing diagnostic descriptions and ensure that patient advocacy groups review and endorse these descriptions, supporting diverse experiences and addressing limitations of traditional scientific standards (e.g. Bueter, 2019).
- **Training in Diagnostic Communication:** Train clinicians not just in making diagnoses but in discussing them with patients. Integrate principles of shared decision-making (Hamann et al., 2003) and respect for patients' desire to know their diagnosis earlier (Perkins et al., 2018), allowing space for alternative formulations such as psychosocial, neurodivergent, or spiritual explanations.
- **Embracing Psychiatry's Unique Role:** Embrace the unique intersection of art, science, and humanities in psychiatry rather than defend against it. Use symptom-based approaches like the Hierarchical Taxonomy of Psychopathology (Kotov et al., 2017) to inform training, steering towards 'relational psychiatry' (Guimón, 2004) that balances humility and confidence in co-creating better practices.
- **Diagnostic Nuance at the Network Level:** Adopt systems approaches like 'Open Dialogue' (Olson et al., 2014), emphasizing uncertainty tolerance and multiple perspectives, allowing patients to construct their narratives. Ensure that principles of epistemic justice guide the ongoing development and revision of psychiatric classification systems like the ICD and DSM.

Though these changes may appear substantial, they reflect a shift from 'doing to' to 'being with,' consistent with horizontalizing power relations and viewing speech and meaning as collaborative enterprises. Such approaches can not only help reduce burnout in providers (e.g. Beale, 2022) but are also more consistent with the emerging evidence base on the complexities of mental health. Lived Experience Practitioners, nearly always experts by experience in power asymmetries, are well-placed to educate practitioners on what epistemic injustice looks like in practice. Texts and videos of real-world consultations can illustrate how what is speakable, hearable, and knowable is co-constructed in dialogue. This training should be comprehensive, covering a range of scenarios—from instances where a patient's narrative is overlooked or pigeonholed into a pre-existing diagnostic category to moments where broader social biases related to race, class, gender, and disability intersect with clinical judgement.

By applying principles of epistemic justice, we can transform the development and revision of major psychiatric classification systems, such as the ICD and DSM, from mere categorization tools into instruments of empowerment. Incorporating objectification, moral agency, trivialization, and narrative agency as navigational tools helps us prioritize a crucial third criterion for diagnoses in addition to reliability and validity: their real-world usefulness. John and Cara's contrasting experiences with depression and BPD underscore the need for these principles. Embracing epistemic justice not only helps us navigate the divisive and damaging diagnostic wars but also centres our focus on the narratives that matter most: those of patients in pain. By doing so, we can move towards a psychiatric practice that honours and uplifts the voices of those it seeks to serve, ultimately creating a more humane and just mental healthcare system.

Acknowledgements I thank the survivor community and especially Mad Twitter and the survivor-led collective 'Recovery in the Bin' for helping me reconsider psychiatric diagnosis beyond a simple pro or con binary perspective. Special thanks to Stefan Priebe and Rose McCabe for keeping me connected to the academic community despite my Mad interludes. My appreciation goes to Lisa Bortolotti and the growing Epistemic Injustice community for work which I hope will genuinely transform power relations in clinical practice.

REFERENCES

Baker, J., & Beazley, P. I. (2022). Judging personality disorder: A systematic review of clinician attitudes and responses to borderline personality disorder. *Journal of Psychiatric Practice®, 28*(4), 275–293.

Beale, C. (2022). Magical thinking and moral injury: Exclusion culture in psychiatry. *BJPsych Bulletin, 46*(1), 16–19.

Beck, A. T., & Alford, B. A. (2009). *Depression: Causes and treatment*. University of Pennsylvania Press.

Bertilsdotter Rosqvist, H., Botha, M., Hens, K., O'Donoghue, S., Pearson, A., & Stenning, A. (2023). Cutting our own keys: New possibilities of neurodivergent storying in research. *Autism, 27*(5), 1235–1244.

British Psychological Society. (2020). *Understanding depression.* Retrieved March 30, 2024, from https://www.bps.org.uk/guideline/understanding-depression

Bueter, A. (2019). Epistemic injustice and psychiatric classification. *Philosophy of Science, 86*(5), 1064–1074.

Cano-Ruiz, P., Sanmartin-Salinas, P., Gómez-Peinado, A., Calero-Mora, C., & Gutiérrez-Rojas, L. (2020). Diagnostic stability in bipolar disorder: A systematic review. *Actas Españolas de Psiquiatría, 48*(1), 28–35.

Chen, S., Boucher, H. C., & Tapias, M. P. (2006). The relational self revealed: Integrative conceptualization and implications for interpersonal life. *Psychological Bulletin, 132*(2), 151.

Crichton, P., Carel, H., & Kidd, I. J. (2017). Epistemic injustice in psychiatry. *BJPsych Bulletin, 41*(2), 65–70.

Cumberlege, J. (2020). *First do no harm: The report of the Independent Medicines and Medical Devices Safety (IMMDS) Review.* Independent Medicines and Medical Devices Safety Review. https://www.immdsreview.org.uk/downloads/IMMDSReview_Web.pdf

Dixon, T. (2023). *The history of emotions: A very short introduction.* Oxford University Press.

Dotson, K. (2011). Tracking epistemic violence, tracking practices of silencing. *Hypatia, 26*(2), 236–257.

Fricker, M. (2007). *Epistemic injustice: Power and the ethics of knowing.* Oxford University Press.

Giedinghagen, A. (2023). The tic in TikTok and (where) all systems go: Mass social media induced illness and Munchausen's by internet as explanatory models for social media associated abnormal illness behavior. *Clinical Child Psychology and Psychiatry, 28*(1), 270–278.

Guimón, J. (2004). *Relational mental health: Beyond evidence-based interventions.* Springer Science & Business Media.

Hamann, J., Leucht, S., & Kissling, W. (2003). Shared decision making in psychiatry. *Acta Psychiatrica Scandinavica, 107*(6), 403–409.

Hawkins, A. A., Furr, R. M., Arnold, E. M., Law, M. K., Mneimne, M., & Fleeson, W. (2014). The structure of borderline personality disorder symptoms: A multi-method, multi-sample examination. *Personality Disorders: Theory, Research, and Treatment, 5*(4), 380.

Henderson, C., & Thornicroft, G. (2009). Stigma and discrimination in mental illness: Time to change. *The Lancet, 373*(9679), 1928–1930.

Herman, J. L. (2015). *Trauma and recovery: The aftermath of violence—From domestic abuse to political terror.* Hachette UK.

Houlders, J. W., Bortolotti, L., & Broome, M. R. (2021). Threats to epistemic agency in young people with unusual experiences and beliefs. *Synthese, 199*(3), 7689–7704.

Insel, T. R. (2014). The NIMH research domain criteria (RDoC) project: Precision medicine for psychiatry. *American Journal of Psychiatry, 171*(4), 395–397.

Jackson, J. (2017). Patronizing depression: Epistemic injustice, stigmatizing attitudes, and the need for empathy. *Journal of Social Philosophy, 48*(3), 359–376.

Kidd, I. J., Spencer, L., & Carel, H. (2023). Epistemic injustice in psychiatric research and practice. *Philosophical Psychology*, 1–29.

Kotov, R., Krueger, R. F., Watson, D., Achenbach, T. M., Althoff, R. R., Bagby, R. M., et al. (2017). The Hierarchical Taxonomy of Psychopathology (HiTOP): A dimensional alternative to traditional nosologies. *Journal of Abnormal Psychology, 126*(4), 454.

Kyratsous, M., & Sanati, A. (2017). Epistemic injustice and responsibility in borderline personality disorder. *Journal of Evaluation in Clinical Practice, 23*(5), 974–980.

Lamb, N., Sibbald, S., & Stirzaker, A. (2018). Shining lights in dark corners of people's lives: Reaching consensus for people with complex mental health difficulties who are given a diagnosis of personality disorder. *Criminal Behaviour and Mental Health, 28*(1), 1–4.

Lam, D. C., Salkovskis, P. M., & Hogg, L. I. (2016). 'Judging a book by its cover': An experimental study of the negative impact of a diagnosis of border-line personality disorder on clinicians' judgements of uncomplicated panic disorder. *British Journal of Clinical Psychology, 55*(3), 253–268.

Langley, L., & Price, E. (2022). *Death by a thousand cuts: Report into the Tees Esk and Wear Valleys NHS Foundation Trust "BPD+" Protocol*. Retrieved March 30, 2024, from https://www.researchgate.net/publication/360939 741_Death_By_A_Thousand_Cuts_Report_into_the_Tees_Esk_and_Wear_V alleys_NHS_Foundation_Trust_BPD_Protocol

Ledford, H. (2013). Psychiatry framework seeks to reform diagnostic doctrine. *Nature*. Retrieved March 30, 2024, from https://doi.org/10.1038/nature. 2013.12972

Linehan, M. M. (1993). *Skills training manual for treating borderline personality disorder*. Guilford Press.

Lomani, J., Alyce, S., Aves, W., Chevous, J., Clayton, E., Conway, D., Donaldson, R., Duffel, A., Ellison, J., Harris, H., Jee, Joran, D., Kitson, S., Newbiggin, K., Perot, C., Richmond, L., Rose, E., Survivors Against PD, Sweeney, A., Taggart, D., Targaryen, Y., Turner, K., Waddingham, R., Walker, T., & Anonymous. (2022). *New ways of supporting child abuse and sexual violence survivors: A social justice call for an innovative commissioning pathway*. Retrieved March 30, 2024, from https://osf.io/svz3w

Lucy's Depression Diary. (2020). *Not an illness? A response to the British Psychological Society report, 'Understanding Depression,' October 2020.* Retrieved March 30, 2024, from https://lucysdepressiondiary.wordpress.com/2020/10/12/not-an-illness-a-response-to-the-british-psychological-society-report-understanding-depression-october-2020/

Mulder, R., & Tyrer, P. (2023). Borderline personality disorder: A spurious condition unsupported by science that should be abandoned. *Journal of the Royal Society of Medicine, 116*(4), 148–150.

National Institute for Mental Health. (2003). *Personality disorder: No longer a diagnosis of exclusion: Policy implementation guidance for the development of services for people with personality disorder.* NIMHE.

Oliffe, J. L., Rossnagel, E., Seidler, Z. E., Kealy, D., Ogrodniczuk, J. S., & Rice, S. M. (2019). Men's depression and suicide. *Current Psychiatry Reports, 21*(10), 1–6.

Olson, M., Seikkula, J., & Ziedonis, D. (2014). The key elements of dialogic practice in open dialogue: Fidelity criteria. *The University of Massachusetts Medical School, 8*, 2017.

Perkins, A., Ridler, J., Browes, D., Peryer, G., Notley, C., & Hackmann, C. (2018). Experiencing mental health diagnosis: A systematic review of service user, clinician, and carer perspectives across clinical settings. *The Lancet Psychiatry, 5*(9), 747–764.

Phillips, J. (2010, December 22). The missing person in the DSM. *Psychiatric Times.* Retrieved March 30, 2024, from https://www.psychiatrictimes.com/view/missing-person-dsm

Recovery in the Bin. (2019, April 3). *RITB position statement on personality disorders (or their euphemisms including complex emotional needs).* Retrieved March 30, 2024, from https://recoveryinthebin.org/2019/04/03/ritb-position-statement-on-personality-disorder/

Russo, J., & Sweeney, A. (Eds.). (2016). *Searching for a rose garden: Challenging psychiatry, fostering mad studies.* PCCS Books.

Sakakibara, E. (2023). Epistemic injustice in the therapeutic relationship in psychiatry. *Theoretical Medicine and Bioethics, 44*(5), 477–502.

Schore, A. N. (2003). *Affect dysregulation and disorders of the self.* Norton Series on Interpersonal Neurobiology. W. W. Norton.

Scrutton, A. P. (2017). Epistemic injustice and mental illness. In *The Routledge handbook of epistemic injustice* (pp. 347–355). Routledge.

Spencer, L., & Carel, H. (2021). 'Isn't everyone a little OCD?' The epistemic harms of wrongful depathologization. *Philosophy of Medicine, 2*(1), 1–18.

Vermetten, E., & Spiegel, D. (2014). Trauma and dissociation: Implications for borderline personality disorder. *Current Psychiatry Reports, 16*, 1–10.

Watts, J. (2017). Testimonial injustice and borderline personality disorder. *Huffington Post*. Retrieved July 25, 2023, from https://www.huffingtonpost.co.uk/dr-jay-watts/testimonial-injusticeand_b_14738494.html

Watts, J. (2019). Problems with the ICD-11 classification of personality disorder. *The Lancet Psychiatry, 6*(6), 461–463.

Watts, J. (2023a). Engendering misunderstanding: Autism and borderline personality disorder. *International Journal of Psychiatry in Clinical Practice, 27*(3), 316–317.

Watts, J. (2023b, Autumn). The personality disorder shield. *New Associations* (41).

White, M., & Epston, D. (1990). *Narrative means to therapeutic ends*. W. W. Norton.

World Health Organization. (2022). *ICD-11 for mortality and morbidity statistics* (11th ed.). Retrieved March 30, 2024, from https://icd.who.int/

Wortham, S. E. (2000). Interactional positioning and narrative self-construction. *Narrative Inquiry, 10*(1), 157–184.

Zimmerman, M., Ellison, W., Young, D., Chelminski, I., & Dalrymple, K. (2015). How many different ways do patients meet the diagnostic criteria for major depressive disorder? *Comprehensive Psychiatry, 56*, 29–34.

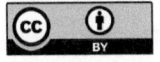

CHAPTER 5

Resisting Perceptions of Patient Untrustworthiness

Eleanor Palafox-Harris⊙

Abstract A beneficial therapeutic relationship between a patient and their clinician requires mutual trust. In order to effectively treat someone, a clinician has to trust the patient's reports of their symptoms, relevant experiences, medical history, and so on. Many psychiatric symptoms do not have physical markers that can be verified by clinical testing, and thus psychiatrists have to accept more on trust than clinicians treating somatic illnesses. However, many psychiatric diagnoses are stereotypically associated with traits that indicate *untrustworthiness* (such as irrationality). In this chapter, I illustrate how psychiatric labels can signal stereotypes of untrustworthiness, and how this can have repercussions in clinical contexts. In particular, I show how perceptions of untrustworthiness cause epistemic injustices by unfairly reducing the perceived epistemic credibility of patients with psychiatric conditions.

Keywords Trustworthiness · Hypervigilance · Mental health patient · Stereotypes · Credibility

E. Palafox-Harris (✉)
Department of Philosophy, University of Birmingham, Birmingham, UK
e-mail: exh692@student.bham.ac.uk

© The Author(s) 2025
L. Bortolotti (ed.), *Epistemic Justice in Mental Healthcare*,
https://doi.org/10.1007/978-3-031-68881-2_5

5.1   TRUST IN CLINICAL ENCOUNTERS

Clinical interactions between patients and practitioners require *trust*.[1] The importance of a patient's trust in their practitioner is plain: the patient has to trust in their clinician's medical expertise, trust their diagnosis and suggested treatment, trust that the clinician has the best interests of the patient at heart, and so on. Numerous studies have explored the importance of patients' trust in their clinicians (for example Hall et al., 2001). However, the clinician's trust in their patients is less researched, but also important. For example, Simone Farrelly and Helen Lester (2014) found that *mutual trust* is important for beneficial relationships between people with psychotic disorders and their clinicians. Rachel Grob and colleagues (2019) suggest that trusting patients carries a number of benefits, including improving diagnosis, improving the doctor-patient relationship, and encouraging mutual trust (as patients are more likely to reciprocate trust in their practitioner if their practitioner has demonstrated their trust in the patient). Furthermore, Wendy Rogers (2002) suggests that a clinician's trust in a patient supports the patient's exercise of autonomy and encourages cooperation between patient and practitioner.

As well as these positive reasons for trusting patients, there are also reasons to *avoid distrusting* patients. Rogers argues that when a clinician wrongly distrusts their patient, the patient is harmed by being *disempowered* (2002: 78). In medical contexts, power dynamics are already asymmetric, as the clinician's presumed expertise and experience gives them 'epistemic privilege' over their patients (Carel & Kidd, 2014). Rogers emphasises that disempowering patients by distrusting them further 'shifts' the unequal power dynamic in favour of the clinician, disadvantaging the patient further (Rogers, 2002: 78). This disempowerment means that 'lack of trust is an unfair burden added to existing burdens of ill health, creating hostility and inhibiting good clinical care' (2002: 80). Consequently, Rogers argues that doctors have a *moral duty* to trust patients. Some important qualifications should be noted here: there are cases where distrust is warranted, and indeed, there are cases

---

[1] Of course, one can draw distinctions between kinds of trust, such as three-place, two-place, and one-place trust. We can also distinguish between thin trust (mere reliance) and thicker accounts of trust. Discussing all of these distinctions and the way they relate to psychiatric healthcare is beyond the scope of this chapter, however, the interested reader could see e.g. Ratcliffe et al. (2014) for a phenomenological study of one-place trust and trauma.

where *trust* might actually be harmful if distrust is appropriate. For example, Rogers suggests that trusting an untrustworthy patient might lead to exploitation of medical resources (2002: 79). Nevertheless, Rogers argues that it is 'morally desirable' for doctors to *aspire to trust* and to adopt a 'trusting attitude' towards patients (2002: 79).

Given the role trust in patients plays in clinical encounters, particularly in psychiatric encounters, we need to consider what makes a patient *trustworthy*, and whether clinicians' perceptions of patient trustworthiness are biased in psychiatric contexts.

The literature on trustworthiness generally stipulates that a person is trustworthy if they meet both an epistemic and a moral criterion. Typically, the epistemic criterion for trustworthiness is labelled *competence* (for example, Hawley, 2019; Hills, 2023; Jones, 2012). That competence is necessary to be deemed trustworthy seems intuitive: I cannot trust what someone is telling me if I do not think they are competent to know what they are talking about. However, how to label the moral criterion for trustworthiness is more contested. Some scholars suggest that trustworthiness is a moral *virtue* (e.g. Hills, 2023; Potter, 2002), whilst others argue against a virtue theory of trustworthiness (e.g. Hawley, 2019; Jones, 2012). Nonetheless, even those who do not conceptualise trustworthiness as moral virtue can accept a moral condition on trustworthiness. Candidates for the moral criterion include *good intentions* (Hawley, 2019), *sincerity* (Fricker, 2007), *goodwill* (Jones, 1996), and *benevolence* (Sperber et al., 2010). For this chapter, I will use *benevolence* to pick out the moral condition for trustworthiness, as benevolence is a broad notion which captures various moral goods, such as moral action (acting benevolently), moral character (being benevolent), and moral intentions (benevolent motivations). However, I take what follows in this chapter to be consistent with any of the proposed moral conditions listed above with some minor adjustment.

There is empirical support for the claim that trustworthiness has an epistemic and moral dimension. The evidence suggests that even children use the perceived competence and benevolence of an informant when making decisions about trustworthiness. For example, Olivier Mascaro and Dan Sperber (2009) found that children as young as three years old prefer the testimony of benevolent informants to malevolent informants. Shiri Einav and Elizabeth Robinson (2011) found that when children reach around four years of age, they discriminate between knowledgeable (competent) informants and merely accurate informants.

The moral and epistemic criteria for trustworthiness might not always (or indeed, often) be equally important for calculations of an individual's trustworthiness. That is, it is highly plausible that the perceived competence of a speaker might be more important than their perceived benevolence in certain situations, and vice versa. For example, Tiffany Barnett White (2005: 147) investigated consumer trust in high-stakes financial decision-making, and found that when decisions are not emotionally difficult, the competence of an informant matters more. However, when the decisions are emotionally difficult, consumers favour benevolent (but still sufficiently competent) informants. In other words, although competence and benevolence are both *necessary* for trust, the moral and epistemic dimensions need not be equally weighted. Nevertheless, a trustworthy speaker must be *sufficiently* competent and benevolent. A trustworthy speaker merits trust. In contrast, an untrustworthy speaker is someone who fails to meet these conditions: someone who is *insufficiently* competent and/or benevolent.[2] An untrustworthy speaker merits distrust. Therefore, we can summarise the conditions for trustworthiness (and untrustworthiness) as follows:

For any speaker, S:
  S merits trust if and only if S is trustworthy.
  S is trustworthy if and only if S is sufficiently competent and sufficiently benevolent.
  If S is untrustworthy, then S merits distrust.
  S is untrustworthy if[3] S is insufficiently competent and/or insufficiently benevolent.

---

[2] There is some middle ground between trustworthiness and untrustworthiness. Someone might fail to be trustworthy because we lack the information to decide how competent or benevolent they are. Additionally, Katherine Hawley points out that there are some subjects who are neither trustworthy nor untrustworthy because neither is a 'suitable category' for them, such as babies (Hawley, 2019: 78–79). However, for this chapter, we can set aside cases where someone does not meet the conditions for trustworthiness due to either lack of information or the unsuitability of trustworthiness categories. As I will show, people with psychiatric labels are perceived as failing to be trustworthy because of the *presence* of information (stereotypes) that indicates untrustworthiness.

[3] Careful readers will notice that the biconditional has been dropped here. This is to account for other factors that might make someone untrustworthy, such as a reputation of being really unreliable.

Throughout the chapter, I talk in terms of *distrust* rather than *mistrust*. This is because in ordinary language the two terms are often used interchangeably, and I follow Katherine Hawley in thinking that the distinction between them is not 'philosophically load-bearing' (Hawley, 2019: 6).

With this work on (a) the importance of trust in the clinical encounter, and (b) the moral and epistemic conditions for trustworthiness in the background, we can return to the topic of distrusting patients with psychiatric diagnoses.

5.2   Psychiatric Labels
and Stereotypes of Untrustworthiness

In healthcare contexts, diagnostic labelling allows healthcare professionals to classify patients. These diagnostic labels carry a number of benefits. For example, for clinicians and researchers, diagnostic labels efficiently summarise a lot of information about a condition, such as symptoms, courses of treatment, and potential prognosis (Garand et al., 2009). Moreover, for patients, diagnostic labelling may facilitate help-seeking behaviour (Yap et al., 2014), and enable people with diagnostic labels to access certain *resources*, both within healthcare contexts (such as medications and treatment programmes, counselling, and so on) and in other social contexts (such as financial aid, support groups, adjustments in the workplace and assistance resources such as mobility aids, care workers, and so on).

Nevertheless, diagnostic labels also 'serve as cues to signal stereotypes' (Garand et al., 2009: 113). As diagnostic labelling allows clinicians to assume that patients are 'generally homogeneous in the underlying nature of the illness' (2009: 113), labelling also facilitates generalisations between people who share the same condition by increasing perceptions of their *groupness* and *homogeneity* (Ben-Zeev et al., 2010: 321). This facilitates stereotyping. For this chapter, I use Katherine Puddifoot's definitions of stereotypes and stereotyping, according to which:

> Stereotype: a social attitude that associates members of some social group more strongly than others with certain trait(s).
>
> Stereotyping: the application of a social attitude that associates members of some social group more strongly than others with certain traits to an individual or individuals who are perceived as a member of the relevant

social group, leading that individual or those individuals to be associated with the trait. (Puddifoot, 2021: 13)

In line with Bruce Link and Jo Phelan's (2001) stigma model, diagnostic labels plausibly facilitate stereotyping by picking out a *difference* (an illness) which is associated with a 'set of undesirable characteristics' (a stereotype). Mental illness is heavily stigmatised, and thus psychiatric labels can signal a number of negative stereotypes (Crichton et al., 2017). Numerous studies investigate the negative effects of psychiatric labels on how people are perceived by others (see for example Magliano et al., 2017) or themselves (e.g. Corrigan et al., 2015). Indeed, the stigma of psychiatric labels is so powerful that some people might avoid seeking mental health care in order to avoid being given a psychiatric label and the stigmatising effects of labelling (Corrigan & Wassel, 2008). For such people, lack of care might mean that their psychiatric condition worsens, and their cognitive and social functioning deteriorates so that they increasingly come to resemble negative stereotypes (a 'self-fulfilling prophecy', as in Kidd & Carel, 2017).

In what follows, I will suggest that the content of many stereotypes about psychiatric diagnoses is in conflict with the criteria for trustworthiness—competence and benevolence—and thus, people with psychiatric labels will struggle to be perceived as meeting the conditions for a trustworthy speaker. I will present two examples of stereotypes relating to particular psychiatric labels (clinical delusion and suicidality), which are in tension with the moral or epistemic conditions for trustworthiness. Although both suicidality and delusion can be *symptoms* of various psychiatric disorders, and not necessarily disorders themselves,[4] I refer to them as *psychiatric labels* because they are socially salient. By this, I mean that both delusion and suicidality are very well-known (if rarely well-understood) symptoms of mental illness, and therefore act as indicators of the presence of mental illness.

Let us take *suicidality* as our first example of a psychiatric label with specific stereotypes that signal untrustworthiness. Suicidality is an umbrella term which encompasses *suicidal behaviours, suicidal ideation,*

---

[4] Delusion *can be* constitutive of a psychiatric disorder (namely, Delusional Disorder), and it has been proposed that the DSM includes Suicidal Behaviour Disorder as a psychiatric disorder in its own right (see e.g. Fehling & Selby, 2021). Nevertheless, delusion and suicidality often occur as symptoms of other disorders, rather than as disorders themselves.

and *suicide*, as well as their sub-concepts (Keefner & Stenvig, 2020: 228). Suicidality is primarily associated with depression and borderline personality disorder but is also a symptom of other psychiatric diagnoses. Research has suggested that although suicidality shares some of the same stereotypes as other mental disorders such as depression, suicidality is also subject to specific stereotype content (Sheehan et al., 2017). Nathalie Oexle and colleagues (2019) suggest that suicidality is stereotyped as '*selfish, attention seeking* and *immoral*' (Oexle et al., 2019: 382, emphasis added). These stereotypical traits straightforwardly conflict with the attribute of *benevolence*, as selfishness, immorality, and so on are clearly not markers of a benevolent informant.

Being stereotyped in this way can negatively affect the attribution of benevolence (and consequently, trustworthiness) in at least two ways. Firstly, being labelled with suicidality pre-emptively *classifies* suicidal patients in a way which precludes the ascription of benevolence, as selfishness and immorality are not compatible with benevolence. This can occur even before an interaction with the patient (before the clinician has formed a perception of them). Secondly, the stereotypes associated with suicidality can deflate *perceptions* of the patient's trustworthiness, as suicidal patients who are stereotyped as selfish, attention-seeking, or immoral would struggle to be perceived as meeting the moral condition for trustworthiness. As the moral criterion is jointly necessary with competence for trustworthiness, the negative traits stereotypically ascribed to suicidal people mean that people labelled with suicidality come out as *untrustworthy* as a result. The negative relationship between suicide and trust is also evident in Corrigan and colleagues' (2017) factor analyses of suicide stigma, in which participants reported feelings of distrust and doubt towards people who attempt suicide. This lends empirical support to my claim that the psychiatric label of suicidality signals untrustworthiness.

Let us now turn to *delusion* as our second example of a psychiatric label with stereotype content that signals untrustworthiness. A clinical delusion is defined in the DSM as a 'fixed belief that is not amenable to change in light of conflicting evidence' (DSM-5, 2013: 87). Clinical delusion can be a symptom of several psychiatric conditions, such as schizophrenia, dementia, and bipolar disorder. Abdi Sanati and Michalis Kyratsous argue that people with delusions are frequently stereotyped as being '*bizarre, incomprehensible,* and *irrational*' (Sanati & Kyratsous, 2015: 484, source emphasis). These traits are in tension with the attribute of *competence*, as bizarreness, irrationality and incomprehensibility are not indicators of a competent informant (Palafox-Harris, 2024). Furthermore, Sanati and Kyratsous argue that for people with delusions, irrationality is 'held as an attribute of the person's general psychic life' (Sanati & Kyratsous, 2015: 484). In other words, people with delusions are not stereotyped as only *locally irrational*, where the irrationality is restricted to the delusion belief(s), but rather *globally irrational*, where irrationality permeates the overall cognition of people with delusions. In a similar way to the label of suicidality, being labelled with delusion pre-emptively classifies patients in a way which precludes the ascription of rationality (and therefore, trustworthiness). Moreover, the stereotypes associated with delusion deflate perceptions of the patients' trustworthiness, as people who are stereotyped as irrational would struggle to be perceived as meeting the epistemic condition for trustworthiness. The psychiatric label for delusion therefore signals untrustworthiness, by triggering stereotypes which conflict with competence.

In summary, we have seen that psychiatric labels are stigmatised and cue negative stereotypes that affect people's perceptions of the person with the psychiatric label. We have also seen how specific stereotype content associated with particular psychiatric labels can signal *untrustworthiness* by conflicting with either the moral or epistemic conditions for trustworthy speakers. Given that untrustworthiness merits distrust, as outlined in §1, the negative stereotyping facilitated by psychiatric labels encourages people to distrust patients with psychiatric diagnoses.

5.3   Distrust and Epistemic Injustice

This distrust of people with psychiatric diagnoses has a number of clinical implications. Mutual trust between a patient and their practitioner is important for certain goods such as improving diagnosis (Grob et al., 2019), hence distrusting patients threatens the attainment of these goods by hindering the development of mutual trust. Moreover, distrust of people with psychiatric diagnoses can create *epistemic injustices*. Epistemic injustice, a notion first articulated by Miranda Fricker (2007), captures instances when someone is harmed in their capacity as a *knower* (Fricker, 2007: 20). This section explores how distrust in patients prompted by psychiatric labelling and stereotypes of untrustworthiness can contribute to different kinds of epistemic injustice (testimonial and hermeneutical) and suggests a few additional considerations related to the nature of distrust and epistemic credibility that complicate the epistemic struggle of being distrusted.

José Medina argues that 'epistemic injustices are rooted in (and deepen) the erosion of trust and the perpetuation of dysfunctional patterns of trust/distrust' (2020: 57). Thus, the notions of trust and distrust, and trustworthiness and untrustworthiness, are intertwined with epistemic injustice (see also Fricker, 2007; Hawley, 2017). This is because many epistemic injustices are intrinsically related to *credibility*, in particular, to unfair underestimations of credibility for marginalised groups (often in contrast to overestimations of credibility for non-marginalised groups [see Medina, 2011]). In paradigmatic cases of *testimonial injustice*, on Fricker's classic account, testimonial injustice occurs when someone sustains an 'identity-prejudicial credibility deficit' (Fricker, 2007: 28). In other words, when a hearer attributes a speaker less credibility than they deserve due to prejudice relating to an aspect of the speaker's social identity, and consequently distrusts their testimony. In Medina's terms, a credibility deficit amounts to 'a very specific kind of trust dysfunction' involving 'misplaced, excessive or malfunctioning *distrust*' (Medina, 2020: 53, source emphasis).

Following John Locke, Karen Jones (1993) argues that the two 'foundations' of credibility are the *trustworthiness* of the testifier and the *plausibility* of their testimony in light of our background beliefs (Jones, 1993: 155). Perceiving a testifier to be untrustworthy thereby undermines their credibility. Fricker suggests that we employ stereotypes when judging a speaker's credibility: 'stereotypes oil the wheels of testimonial exchange' (2007: 32) because stereotypes can act as heuristic aids which bypass the cognitively costly process of accurately evaluating an individual's credibility in a certain context. Nevertheless, these stereotypes—whilst cognitively cheap and therefore efficient means of assessing credibility— also enable *bias*. Fricker argues that prejudicial stereotypes *distort* the credibility judgements we make by biasing our perceptions of a speaker and causing credibility deficits (Fricker, 2007: 36). Therefore, we can see the role of psychiatric labelling and negative stereotypes in bringing about testimonial injustices:

1. A psychiatric label activates stereotypes that signal untrustworthiness (e.g. irrationality, incompetence).
2. This causes the speaker to be perceived as untrustworthy; they sustain a *credibility deficit*.

3. Consequently, the speaker's testimony is treated with suspicion or distrust.

When the credibility deficit sustained by the speaker is ill-grounded, for example, if it was caused by a biased perception of credibility based on unfair stereotypes, then the speaker suffers a testimonial injustice when their testimony is distrusted. Viewed as a trust *dysfunction*, the patients in such cases experience unwarranted (hence excessive) distrust. In this way, psychiatric labelling and stereotypes of untrustworthiness generate testimonial injustices by prompting people (including clinicians and other healthcare practitioners) to unfairly underestimate the epistemic credibility of people with psychiatric diagnoses.

Distrusting patients with psychiatric diagnoses can also contribute to *hermeneutical injustices*. On Fricker's classic account, hermeneutical injustice occurs when 'a gap in collective interpretive resources puts someone at an unfair disadvantage when it comes to making sense of their social experience' (Fricker, 2007: 1). In other words, hermeneutical injustices occur when someone's ability to interpret or articulate an aspect of their social experience is unjustly undermined, or when their capacity to participate in meaning-making and meaning-sharing practices faces 'unfair obstacles' (Medina, 2020: 55). Medina suggests that hermeneutical injustices can be thought of as 'dysfunctions of hermeneutical trust/distrust' (Medina, 2020: 55). This might take the form of dysfunctional relations of trust and distrust between a hermeneutical community and the communicators within it (a trust dysfunction at the *collective level*), and/or it might involve dysfunctions that are maintained by the unjust epistemic practices of individuals (a trust dysfunction at the *interpersonal level*) (Medina, 2020: 56). I will now consider some of the ways in which patients with psychiatric diagnoses might experience hermeneutical injustice, and consider how we can interpret these as dysfunctions in patterns of trust and distrust.

People with psychiatric diagnoses can experience hermeneutical injustice as a result of epistemic asymmetries and power imbalances within clinical contexts. Havi Carel and Ian James Kidd argue that healthcare professionals typically experience *epistemic privilege* in healthcare settings on the basis of their medical training and expertise (Carel & Kidd, 2014: 534–535). One important way that this epistemic privilege contributes to hermeneutical injustice is through *language*. Clinicians are epistemically privileged in setting the authoritative language for medicine, such as the terms for symptoms, the standards of intelligibility, and diagnostic labels (Carel & Kidd, 2014: 535–536). This means that the interpretative resources available for patients to make sense of articulate and their experiences of illness are typically those made by or for healthcare professionals, rather than by people with personal experience of the illness. For some patients, these resources might not adequately capture their experiences or could distort or occlude important aspects of them. However, given the assumed authority of clinical terms and concepts, describing ill-health in non-medicalised language risks not being taken seriously in clinical contexts. In this way, Kristen Steslow argues that '[t]he patient loses her ability to speak with authority except to the extent that her language conforms to the standard medical discourse' (Steslow, 2010: 30). Steslow, who has experienced involuntary psychiatric detention, argues that making herself intelligible to the psychiatric team required adopting their clinical language, and in so doing, 'forsaking the uniqueness of [her] own perspective, understanding, and expression' (2010: 30).

To put this in terms of a hermeneutical trust/distrust dysfunction, in clinical interaction, there is dysfunctional level of trust ascribed to medical language and clinician expertise over and above the patient's own interpretative resources and personal experience. The hermeneutical resources of the privileged group (in this case, clinicians and other healthcare professionals, and the medical institution as a whole) are considered more trustworthy than the hermeneutical resources of patients. Distrusting patients' own language for expressing their experiences of ill-health—by dismissing it as unintelligible, irrelevant, too emotional, or simply inferior to clinical descriptors—bolsters the epistemic authority of medical language and the epistemic privilege of clinicians.

Moreover, the process of psychiatric diagnosis can itself give rise to hermeneutical injustices. Anastasia Scrutton argues that in a medical interview, a patient's experiences can be 'forced into an existing mould' (Scrutton, 2017: 348). In other words, the subjective experiences of the patient are reduced into symptoms of rigid, pre-existing diagnostic categories—ones designed not to advance the self-understanding of the patient but to advance medical-epistemic goals. Scrutton suggests that psychiatric diagnosis effectively *monopolises* how patient experiences are interpreted, as 'the ability to interpret the experience correctly is perceived as lying with the physician' (2017: 348), and this medical perspective is considered authoritative. This problematically excludes other interpretations of the patient's experience, including the patient's own personally relevant interpretation. Of course, *relevance* is a complicated and context-sensitive notion (see Hookway, 2010 for discussion). Nevertheless, for psychiatric conditions, the patient's own meaning-making often matters. Psychiatric labelling therefore contributes to hermeneutical injustices by forcing' rich subjective experiences into fixed diagnostic criteria and thereby overriding the non-medicalised interpretations of those experiences which might be personally meaningful for the patient. The dysfunction in hermeneutical trust/distrust at work here can be interpreted as a dysfunction in the levels of trust accorded to the clinical interpretation compared to the personal interpretation, where one (the clinical diagnosis) is regarded as correct and authoritative, to the exclusion of the other. This is not to say that the patient's interpretation of their experience should necessarily be considered *equally* authoritative, but rather merely to highlight how the diagnostic process, with its pre-defined categories and labels, leaves little room for the patient's personal interpretations and meanings which might not fit those diagnostic 'moulds'.

In summary, we have seen that distrusting patients with psychiatric diagnoses can facilitate, create, or contribute to a variety of epistemic injustices. Finally, I will highlight three considerations which further complicate the precarious epistemic status of people who sustain credibility deficits: the self-fulfilling aspect of distrust, distrust spillover, and the difficulty of recovering lost epistemic status. Firstly, Jones (among others) argues that distrust is *self-fulfilling* (1993; also 2019). That is, once we are suspicious of a speaker, our distrust becomes an interpretational scheme through which we judge their testimony: 'we interpret her story through the lens of our distrust' (Jones, 1993: 159). This encourages us to seek out evidence of the speaker's untrustworthiness:

> [Distrust] leads us to look for signs of deception, irrationality or incompetence and thus leads us to seek out evidence of inconsistencies, to magnify those we suppose ourselves to have found, and to focus on them in our assessment of a story as a whole. (Jones, 1993: 159)

Distrust *distorts* our interpretation of a testifier and of their testimony; we interpret them in ways which confirm our initial distrust (D'Cruz,

2020: 48). In this way, distrust is self-fulfilling for the *person doing the distrusting*.

We can see how the self-fulfilling aspect of distrust can generate testimonial injustices in the healthcare contexts this volume is interested in. Once a clinician is suspicious of a patient (regarding their capacity as an epistemic agent), for example, due to stereotypes of untrustworthiness associated with their psychiatric label, then their initial distrust plausibly distorts their interpretations of the patient's trustworthiness and the trustworthiness of their testimony, leading the clinician to discount their testimony and/or truncate the patient's epistemic participation in the clinical interaction. For example, suppose a patient has been diagnosed with delusion. We have seen that people with delusions are stereotypically ascribed *irrationality*, which conflicts with the epistemic criterion for being trustworthy. This stereotype might cause a clinician to make a pre-judgement that the patient is irrational (and therefore an untrustworthy testifier). Plausibly, due to the self-confirming nature of distrust, the clinician's initial pre-judgement of irrationality becomes an interpretational scheme through which the patient's testimony is judged, biasing the clinician's assessment. This might mean that the patient's testimony is unfairly discounted as being irrational, or that the patient's epistemic participation in the clinical interaction—for example, their role in decision-making, their ability to ask questions or offer alternative interpretations and narratives—is unfairly undermined or restricted.

A consequence of interpreting the patient's testimony through the 'lens of distrust' is that it prevents the clinician from appropriately *updating* their perception of the patient. In seeking confirmation of untrustworthiness or irrationality, distrust obscures counterevidence of trustworthiness and competence: we become 'insensible to signals that others are trustworthy' (D'Cruz, 2020: 48). A consideration of the self-fulfilling aspect of distrust in relation to clinical interaction sheds light on some of the complexities of epistemic injustice. Firstly, it shows that epistemic injustices can arise *prior to*, as well as during, an individual clinical interaction (see Hookway, 2010 on pre-emptive testimonial injustices). Secondly, it shows that epistemic injustices can arise not only from an unfair perception of a patient as untrustworthy, but also from a failure to *update* this perception over time. This means that epistemic injustices are not only 'individual episodic failures' but are instead 'dynamical and diachronic' (Kidd et al., 2023), meaning they can arise at multiple stages of the clinical encounter from a variety of epistemically unjust practices.

Moreover, Jason D'Cruz (2020) suggests that distrust can also be self-fulfilling for the *person being distrusted*. D'Cruz argues that unwarranted distrust 'eats away' at a person's trustworthiness (2020: 47). This is because being unfairly distrusted might erode the person's motivation to be trustworthy. If the person who is distrusted feels that it is impossible to vindicate themselves in the eyes of those who distrust them, then they 'will lack the incentive to seek esteem' (D'Cruz, 2020: 47). As a result, the person who is unfairly distrusted will also miss the opportunity to prove their trustworthiness to *themselves*, which will prevent them from cultivating a 'self-concept' of themselves as a trustworthy person (D'Cruz, 2020: 47). In these ways, distrust reinforces untrustworthiness by eroding a person's motivation to be trustworthy and to prove their trustworthiness to others and to themselves, and consequently affects their self-perception. Distrust can also reinforce *self-stigma*, as the distrusted person might come to accept stereotypes of untrustworthiness and apply them to themselves, resulting in decreased self-esteem, self-efficacy, and self-respect (in line with Corrigan et al., 2015).

We can imagine that a patient with a psychiatric diagnosis who is unfairly distrusted by their practitioner might feel like trying to prove their trustworthiness is futile, particularly because the power imbalances and epistemic asymmetry that exist between patient and their practitioner mean that the practitioner's clinical perspective is assumed to be *authoritative*, or at least treated as authoritative, and therefore difficult for a patient to challenge. Moreover, a patient challenging a clinician's opinion might be interpreted uncharitably as being *uncooperative*. Being perceived as uncooperative can have serious implications in psychiatric healthcare contexts. For example, Irina Georgieva and colleagues (2012) found that patient uncooperativeness 'significantly predicted the use of coercive measures on an acute psychiatric ward' (Georgieva et al., 2012: 419). Therefore, testimony which challenges the clinician's interpretation (including their interpretation of the patient's trustworthiness) might be *risky* for a patient with a psychiatric diagnosis. This might lead a patient to silence their own testimony, as in *testimonial smothering* (Dotson, 2011).

Secondly, distrust is prone to *spillover* (Jones, 2013: 195). Spillover occurs 'when an attitude loses focus on its original target and spreads to neighbouring targets' (Jones, 2013: 195). Jones argues that distrust 'readily falsely generalises' (2013: 196). Distrust spillover happens when someone's distrust of an individual is generalised to other related targets (such as people of the same race, gender, religion, or other social group).

For example, suppose someone judges an individual with a foreign accent to be untrustworthy. Their distrust of a particular person with a foreign accent might falsely generalise to other people with foreign accents. D'Cruz writes that it is 'distressingly familiar how this aspect of distrust can be leveraged by those seeking to stoke distrust of marginalized groups such as refugees and asylum seekers by fixating on dramatic but unrepresentative cases' (2020: 48). In a similar way, we can imagine that someone who distrusts an individual with a psychiatric diagnosis might generalise untrustworthiness to others with that psychiatric diagnosis, particularly given the negative portrayals of people with mental illness in the mass media. Through spillover, distrust in members of a certain group is perpetuates and becomes entrenched.

A third factor which makes having diminished epistemic status particularly perilous is the difficulty of repairing epistemic credibility once it is lost. People who sustain credibility deficits, such as patients with psychiatric diagnoses, can suffer a 'lock-out' effect (Palafox-Harris, 2024) whereby they are prevented from engaging in the epistemic practices that could repair their epistemic status. Cynthia Townley (2011) suggests that having low epistemic credibility is similar to suffering from 'Cassandra's Curse' from Greek Mythology. In the myth, Cassandra receives the gift of prophecy but is cursed by the god Apollo so that no-one will believe her claims. Cassandra cannot defend her prophecies because she is fully excluded from participating in the epistemic community on the basis of her low credibility (Townley, 2011: 44–45). For Cassandra, no amount of truth-telling will restore her epistemic credibility: 'Everything she knows and claims is tarred with the same brush' (2011: 44). Similarly, those who are ascribed low epistemic credibility (such as patients with psychiatric diagnoses) will struggle to repair their status as *knowers*, because they will be unable to successfully prove their trustworthiness and defend their testimony to those who have already judged them to be untrustworthy informants.

A study Toby Pilditch and colleagues (2020) provides empirical support for the existence of a phenomenon like the lock-out effect. Pilditch and colleagues found that 'sources accompanied by low trust cues not only have truthful communications rejected, but have their low trust penalized even further' (Pilditch et al., 2020: 1). This means that once someone is judged as untrustworthy, their subsequent truthful claims are rejected and the fact that their claims are true does not restore their epistemic credibility. If we apply these findings to patients with psychiatric diagnoses, we can see reason to think that a person with a psychiatric diagnosis who is perceived as untrustworthy (for example due to stereotypically ascribed irrationality) would find it difficult to repair their status as a credible epistemic agent, even when their subsequent testimony is rational and competent.

5.4   Beyond Distrust and Blind Trust

In this chapter, I have explored how psychiatric labelling can signal stereotypes such as irrationality and incompetence which are in tension with the criteria for trustworthiness. I have suggested that people with psychiatric diagnoses will struggle to be perceived as trustworthy informants in light of these negative stereotypes, leading them to be unfairly distrusted. Rogers advises that distrusting patients is 'an unfair burden added to existing burdens of ill health' (2002: 80). This distrust is even more burdensome when we consider that distrust is often self-fulfilling for both the one doing the distrusting (the practitioner) and the one being distrusted (the patient), and that lost epistemic credibility is incredibly difficult to regain. Moreover, distrust might spillover from the target (a particular patient with a psychiatric diagnosis) to 'neighbouring targets' (such as other people with the same diagnosis), thereby entrenching distrust in patients and burdening others as well. Distrusting patients with psychiatric diagnoses can create and sustain testimonial and hermeneutical injustices in clinical interactions.

Importantly, in highlighting the role psychiatric labelling and stereotypes of untrustworthiness can play in bringing about epistemic injustices, I do not mean to suggest that distrusting patients with psychiatric diagnoses always constitutes epistemic injustice. There are many instances where distrust of a patient can be appropriate, when the clinician's distrust is well-grounded and unbiased. Elizabeth Barnes points out that patient testimony often involves 'a complex mix of claims' (2023: 654), including claims about the patient's subjective experience of their illness and claims about the aetiology of their illness (2023: 660). Whilst, all else being equal, patients should be trusted about their subjective experience of illness, Barnes argues that clinicians *should not* trust patients about claims relating to the objective parameters of their illness (2023: 663).

Thus, this chapter should not be read as advocating for *blind trust* in patients with psychiatric diagnoses. Instead, it aims to elucidate how psychiatric labelling and stereotypes of untrustworthiness can unfairly distort a hearer's perception of patients, leading them to be pre-emptively judged as untrustworthy, and to experience a level of distrust that is unwarranted. To adopt Medina's (2020) terminology, it is about recognising *dysfunctions* in trust and distrust patterns within psychiatry. Avoiding the epistemic injustices explored in the final section requires a sensitivity to the possibility that perceptions of patient trustworthiness are biased by the negative stereotypes signalled by psychiatric labels, in order to redress the testimonial and hermeneutical trust/distrust dysfunctions that occur in clinical interactions.

Acknowledgements I gratefully acknowledge funding from the AHRC Midlands4Cities Doctoral Training Partnership. Thanks also to Lisa Bortolotti, Ema Sullivan-Bissett, and Ian James Kidd for their helpful feedback on this chapter.

References

American Psychiatric Association. (2013). *Diagnostic and statistical manual of mental disorders: DSM-5* (5th ed.). American Psychiatric Publishing.

Barnes, E. (2023). Trust, distrust, and 'medical gaslighting.' *The Philosophical Quarterly, 73*(3), 649–676.

Barnett White, T. (2005). Consumer trust and advice acceptance: The moderating roles of benevolence, expertise, and negative emotions. *Journal of Consumer Psychology, 15*(2), 141–148.

Ben-Zeev, D., Young, M. A., & Corrigan, P. W. (2010). DSM-V and the stigma of mental illness. *Journal of Mental Health, 19*(4), 318–327.

Carel, H., & Kidd, I. J. (2014). Epistemic injustice in healthcare: A philosophical analysis. *Medicine, Health Care and Philosophy, 17*, 529–540.

Corrigan, P. W., Bink, A. B., Schmidt, A., Jones, N., & Rüsch, N. (2015). What is the impact of self-stigma? Loss of self-respect and the "why try" effect. *Journal of Mental Health, 25*(1), 10–15.

Corrigan, P. W., Sheehan, L., & Al-Khouja, M. A. (2017). Making sense of the public stigma of suicide: Factor analyses of its stereotypes, prejudices, and discriminations. *Crisis, 38*(5), 351–359.

Corrigan, P. W., & Wassel, A. (2008). Understanding and Influencing the Stigma of Mental Illness. *Journal of Psychosocial Nursing and Mental Health Services, 46(1)*, 42–48.

Crichton, P., Carel, H., & Kidd, I. J. (2017). Epistemic injustice in psychiatry. *BJPsych Bulletin, 41*, 65–70.

D'Cruz, J. (2020). Trust and distrust. In J. Simon (Ed.), *The Routledge handbook of trust and philosophy* (pp. 41–51). Routledge.

Dotson, K. (2011). Tracking epistemic violence, tracking practices of silencing. *Hypatia, 26(2)*, 236–257.

Einav, S., & Robinson, E. J. (2011). When being right is not enough: Four-year-olds distinguish knowledgeable informants from merely accurate informants. *Psychological Science, 22*(10), 1250–1253.

Farrelly, S., & Lester, H. (2014). Therapeutic relationships between mental health service users with psychotic disorders and their clinicians: A critical interpretive synthesis. *Health and Social Care in the Community, 22*(5), 449–460.

Fehling, K. B., & Selby, E. A. (2021). Suicide in DSM-5: Current evidence for the proposed suicide behavior disorder and other possible improvements. *Frontiers in Psychiatry, 11*, 499980.

Fricker, M. (2007). *Epistemic injustice: Power and the ethics of knowing*. Oxford University Press.

Garand, L., Lingler, J. H., Conner, K. O., & Dew, M. A. (2009). Diagnostic labels, stigma, and participation in research related to dementia and mild cognitive impairment. *Research Is Gerontological Nursing, 2*(2), 112–121.

Georgieva, I., Vesselinov, R., & Mulder, C. L. (2012). Early detection of risk factors for seclusion and restraint: A prospective study. *Early Intervention in Psychiatry, 6*, 415–422.

Grob, R., Darien, G., & Meyers, D. (2019). Why physicians should trust in patients. *JAMA, 321*(14), 1347–1348.

Hall, M. A., Dugan, E., Zheng, B., & Mishra, A. N. (2001). Trust in physicians and medical institutions: What is it, can it be measured, and does it matter? *The Milbank Quarterly, 79*(4), 613–639.

Hawley, K. (2017). Trust, distrust, and epistemic injustice. In I. J. Kidd, J. Medina, & G. Pohlhaus (Eds.), *The Routledge handbook of epistemic injustice* (pp. 69–78). Routledge.

Hawley, K. (2019). *How to be trustworthy*. Oxford University Press.

Hills, A. (2023). Trustworthiness, responsibility and virtue. *The Philosophical Quarterly, 73*(3), 743–761.

Hookway, C. (2010). Some varieties of epistemic injustice: Reflections on Fricker. *Episteme, 7*(2), 151–163.

Jones, K. (1993). The politics of credibility. In L. Antony & C. Witt (Eds.), *A mind of one's own: Feminist essays on reason and objectivity* (pp. 154–176). Routledge.

Jones, K. (1996). Trust as an Affective Attitude. *Ethics, 107*(1), 4–25.

Jones, K. (2012). Trustworthiness. *Ethics, 123*, 61–85.

Jones, K. (2013). Distrusting the trustworthy. In D. Archard, M. Deveaux, N. Manson, & D. Weinstock (Eds.), *Reading Onora O'Neill* (pp. 186–198). Routledge.

Jones, K. (2019). Trust, distrust, and affective looping. *Philosophical Studies, 176,* 955–968.

Keefner, T. P., & Stenvig, T. (2020). Suicidality: An evolutionary concept analysis. *Issues in Mental Health Nursing, 42*(3), 227–238.

Kidd, I. J., & Carel, H. (2017). Epistemic injustice and illness. *Journal of Applied Philosophy, 34*(2), 172–190.

Kidd, I. J., Spencer, L., & Harris, E. (2023). Epistemic injustice should matter to psychiatrists. *Philosophy of Medicine, 4*(1), 1–4.

Link, B. G., & Phelan, J. C. (2001). Conceptualizing stigma. *Annual Review of Sociology, 27,* 363–385.

Magliano, L., Strino, A., Punzo, R., Acone, R., Affuso, G. & Read J. (2017). Effects of the diagnostic label 'schizophrenia' actively used or passively accepted on general practitioners' views of this disorder. *International Journal of Social Psychiatry, 63(3),* 224–234.

Mascaro, O., & Sperber, D. (2009). The moral, epistemic, and mindreading components of children's vigilance towards deception. *Cognition, 112,* 367–380.

Medina, J. (2011). The relevance of credibility excess in a proportional view of epistemic injustice: Differential epistemic authority and the social imaginary. *Social Epistemology, 25*(1), 15–35.

Medina, J. (2020). Trust and epistemic injustice. In J. Simon (Ed.), *The Routledge handbook of trust and philosophy* (pp. 52–63). Routledge.

Oexle, N., Herrmann, K., Staiger, T., Sheehan, L., Rüsch, N., & Krumm, S. (2019). Stigma and suicidality among suicide attempt survivors: A qualitative study. *Death Studies, 43*(6), 381–388.

Palafox-Harris, E. (2024). Delusion and epistemic injustice. In E. Sullivan-Bissett (Ed.), *The Routledge handbook of the philosophy of delusion.* Routledge.

Pilditch, T. D., Madsen, J. K., & Custers, R. (2020). False prophets and Cassandra's curse: The role of credibility in belief updating. *Acta Psychologica, 202*(102956), 1–12.

Potter, N. N. (2002). *How can I be trusted? A virtue theory of trustworthiness.* Rowman & Littlefield.

Puddifoot, K. (2021). *How stereotypes deceive us.* Oxford University Press.

Ratcliffe, M., Ruddell, M., & Smith, B. (2014). What is "a sense of foreshortened future?" A phenomenological study of trauma, trust, and time. *Frontiers in Psychology, 5,* 1026.

Rogers, W. A. (2002). Is there a moral duty for doctors to trust patients? *Journal of Medical Ethics, 28,* 77–80.

Sanati, A., & Kyratsous, M. (2015). Epistemic injustice in assessment of delusions. *Journal of Evaluation of Clinical Practice, 21*(3), 479–485.

Scrutton, A. (2017). Epistemic injustice and mental illness. In I. J. Kidd, J. Medina, & G. Pohlhaus (Eds.), *The Routledge Handbook of Epistemic Injustice* (pp. 347–355). Routledge.

Sheehan, L., Dubke, R., & Corrigan, P. W. (2017). The specificity of public stigma: A comparison of suicide and depression-related stigma. *Psychiatry Research, 256,* 40–45.

Sperber, D., Clément, F., Heintz, C., Mascaro, O., Mercier, H., Origgi, G., & Wilson, D. (2010). Epistemic vigilance. *Mind & Language, 25,* 359–393.

Steslow, K. (2010). Metaphors in Our Mouths: The Silencing of the Psychiatric Patient. *Hastings Center Report, 40*(4), 30–33.

Townley, C. (2011). *A defense of ignorance: Its value for knowers and roles in feminist and social epistemologies.* Lexington Books.

Yap, M. B. H., Reavley, N. J., & Jorm, A. F. (2014). The associations between psychiatric label use and young people's help-seeking preferences: Results from an Australian National Survey. *Epidemiology and Psychiatric Sciences, 23,* 51–59.

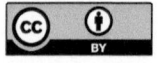

CHAPTER 6

Preserving Dignity and Epistemic Justice in Palliative Care for Patients with Serious Mental Health Problems

Luigi Grassi◉, Marco Cruciata, Martino Belvederi Murri◉, Federica Folesani◉, and Rosangela Caruso◉

Abstract Dignity and preservation of dignity have emerged as a central and mandatory aim to pursue in all the areas of medicine, including palliative care. People with severe mental disorders (SMI) who are at the end of life pose further challenges because of the problem of stigma, which is intrinsically imbued in palliative care, as well as of other the variables including marginalization, alienation, and epistemic injustice typically associated with mental illness and psychiatry. A person-centred approach, which promotes a medicine *of* the person, *for* the person, *by* the person, and *with* the person, can increase the sense of personal dignity, as the other side of stigma, and epistemic justice for patients with SMI who are at the end of life. Dignity-oriented intervention, such as Dignity Therapy, can also be applied in palliative care settings for people with SMI

L. Grassi (✉) · M. Cruciata · M. Belvederi Murri · F. Folesani · R. Caruso
Institute of Psychiatry, Department of Neuroscience and Rehabilitation,
University of Ferrara, Ferrara, Italy
e-mail: luigi.grassi@unife.it

© The Author(s) 2025
L. Bortolotti (ed.), *Epistemic Justice in Mental Healthcare*,
https://doi.org/10.1007/978-3-031-68881-2_6

105

with the aim to offer them an opportunity to reflect upon crucial existential and relational issues, to review aspects of their lives and of self, and to help in preparing a legacy of memories, words of love and wisdom with significant others.

Keywords Dignity · Palliative care · Psychiatry · Palliative psychiatry · Stigma · Discrimination

6.1   AN INTRODUCTION TO DIGNITY

Dignity, as a core tenant of human life and human rights, has been studied by many different perspectives including philosophy, ethics, law, sociology, and medicine. In Greek, dignity (ἀρετή, arête) describes the concept of "virtue" or "excellence" which encompasses a wide range of qualities, such as moral, intellectual, as well as physical excellence. The current use of the word dignity is derived from the Latin *decus* (ornament, distinction, honour, glory, but also worthiness of honour and esteem) and *dignitas,* which is *"an individual or group's sense of self-respect and self-worth, physical and psychological integrity and empowerment"* (Lebech, 2009; Rosen, 2012). Both Greek and Latin concepts emphasize the importance of treating individuals with respect, compassion, and understanding, regardless of their social status, health, or abilities.

From that time, the philosophical Kantian tradition states that dignity is *"an inviolable property of all human beings, which gives the possessor the right never to be treated simply as a mean, but always at the same time as an end, because of its ultimate moral worth"* (Spiegelberg, 1971). Although, some scholars, such as Macklin (2003) provocatively consider dignity a useless concept, stating that dignity is simply not different from respect and personal autonomy, when applied to medical contexts, dignity and preservation of dignity have emerged as a central and mandatory aim to pursue in healthcare. Dignity-preserving care and interventions preserving dignity in medicine have attracted the attention of psychooncology, psychosocial, and psychiatric literature over the last twenty years. This responds to the need for changing the objectifying, biotechnological approach of modern medicine into a more dignified and subjective approach (Grassi et al., 2024). In their model, Chochinov (2002, 2006) and Chochinov et al. (2002) indicate that dignity in the context of palliative care consists of three primary dimensions: (i) *illness-related concerns* (e.g., concerns related to symptoms of physical and psychological distress, and functional capacity) that threaten or impinge on the individual sense of dignity; (ii) *dignity-conserving perspectives and practices* (e.g., continuity of the self, role preservation, maintenance of pride, hopefulness); and (iii) *social aspects of dignity* (e.g., social support, burden to others, aftermath concerns), which define the relationship between patients and their healthcare professionals.

In a review of 9 qualitative and 13 quantitative studies, aspects of dignity have been explicitly identified by the patients themselves who considered this dimension as determined by the overlapping between several components (e.g., autonomy, respect, acceptance), including spiritual and faith issues (Xiao et al., 2021). It is a fact that there is a myriad of ways in which patients' dignity can be compromised in the medical setting, including psychiatry and palliative care. These include rudeness, indifference, condescension, dismissal, disregard, intrusion, objectification, restriction, labelling, contempt, discrimination, revulsion, and deprivation, from the part of healthcare professionals (Grassi et al., 2019). On the other hand, the structure of the healthcare system can cause many professionals experience increasing demands and caseloads, inadequate resources, and uncertainty about the best way to approach their work which, in turn, determine a series of *"assaults on human dignity, intrinsic as well as attributed, that are taken for granted in the bureaucratic, commercialized, and impersonal places that hospitals have, all too often, become"*, as Pellegrino (2008) pungently described.

What Pellegrino underlines is markedly connected with the concept of epistemic injustice that also is gradually emerging in medicine, including psychiatry (Ritunnano, 2022). Epistemic injustice has been introduced by Fricker (2007) who underlined two forms of it. Testimonial injustice describes situations where knowledge, experiences, and contributions of people are not believed because of negative stereotypes attached to their social group, identity, or status. A different form is hermeneutic injustice which is represented by the inability of people to express their experience because of a lack of common language. This is particularly evident in patients with severe psychiatric disorders in whom the problem is not education or lack of property in language, but an epistemic marginalization caused by the difficulty to be understood by others because of the symptoms of mental illness, such as delusions, distortions of reality test, or disturbance of thought process and perception. Therefore, loss of dignity and non-dignity experiences among patients with serious mental illnesses (SMI), such as schizophrenia, bipolar, and mood disorders, are imbued by epistemic injustice and inequity that should be constantly monitored and solved as problems negatively influencing both the quality of care and the quality of patients' life.

This is particularly evident when people with SMI become affected by somatic disorders, especially when in an advanced phase palliative care is necessary (Lawrence & Kisely, 2010). Palliative and end-of-life interventions are themselves at risk of not providing dignity-oriented care, because of both inequalities and epistemic injustice, again for the common prejudices about palliative care—palliation as futile and useless in terms of healing—and misinformation about the discipline—for instance, care for imminent dying and use of opioids as a way to favour substance abuse (Alcalde & Zimmermann, 2022; Formagini et al., 2022; Shen & Wellman, 2019).

In this chapter, we will first discuss the problem of dignity in people with SMI. Then we will focus attention on the problem of dignity at the end of life, examining possible interventions to develop a person-centred and dignified approach.

6.2   Dignity and Stigma Among People with SMI

The World Health Organization (WHO) has repeatedly highlighted the importance of promoting principles such as social justice, equality, and dignity for people affected by mental disorders with the aim to end their marginalization and social disenfranchisement (as in the WHO Mental Health Action Plan 2013–2030). Respect for the inherent human dignity should also be part of developing policies, plans, and services in the area of mental health. The WHO affirms that living a life with dignity stems from the respect of basic human rights, such as freedom from violence and abuse; freedom from discrimination; autonomy and self-determination; inclusion in community life; and participation in policy making. This is therefore related to dignity as the individual's inherent value and worth, and to the need for respect, recognition, self-worth and ability to make choices.

Despite these efforts, a contrasting public attitude exists towards people with SMI and stigma is one of the most significant and hard to eradicate problems in psychiatry (Corrigan et al., 2003; Corrigan &

Watson, 2002; Mestdagh & Hansen, 2014). Stereotypes, prejudice, and discrimination continue to exist for people with SMI, not only for relational encounters in daily life, but also in the healthcare setting and among healthcare providers, with obvious negative consequences on patients' dignity (Bhugra et al., 2016; Livingston & Boyd, 2010).

It is important to separate several forms of stigma: *self-stigma* is the internalization of public stigma and prejudices influencing an individual's self-conception with secondary feelings of shame, anger, hopelessness, or despair; *social stigma* (public and institutional stigma) refers to both a set of social negative attitudes and beliefs that motivate individuals to fear, reject, avoid, and discriminate against people with mental illness and the organizational policies or a culture of negative attitudes and beliefs about mental illness (Gray, 2002; Hinshaw & Stier, 2008). On the same premises, lack of interest in the experience of individuals affected by mental illness can reduce the possibility for them to narrate and offer an interpretation of their illness. It can also dismiss the person as someone who does not have the right to be respected in terms of reasoning, believing, and knowing activities (Drożdżowicz, 2021, Slack & Barclay, 2023). All these aspects are again prominent dimensions of epistemic injustice which may be involved in the clinical encounter. Receiving a psychiatric diagnosis (Hassall, 2024; Sakakibara, 2023) and being reductively objectified by pre-determined criteria based on symptoms rather than on the personal representation of the symptoms are evident manifestations of epistemic injustice (Spencer, 2023).

The concept of stigma—and by extension epistemic injustice—is related to that of dignity, as the other side of the same coin. In fact, as it is for stigma, dignity can be similarly conceived as formed by an *intrinsic component* (or *self-dignity*), that is, the worth, stature, or value that human beings have simply because they are human; and an *attributed component* (or *social dignity*), that is, the worth, stature, or value that human beings confer upon others by acts of affirmation. Jacobson (2007) and Barclay (2016) refer to a *dignity-of-self* (the dignity we attach to ourselves as integrated and autonomous persons) and a *dignity-in-relation* (the dignity that we perceive or do not perceive within interpersonal relationships).

On these bases, Grassi (manuscript in preparation) and Grassi and Chochinov (2024) have developed a model in which stigma and dignity are mutually interrelated. What is done to reduce stigma in mental health settings results in an increase of dignity and what facilitates stigma results in a non-dignity experience for patients. The literature regarding the relationship between dignity and stigma among people with psychiatric disorders supports the notion that dignity means to be treated as an equal human being. A lack of compassion in healthcare settings results in patient suffering from feeling inferior and stigmatized (Burns, 2009; Skorpen et al., 2014; Whitley & Campbell, 2014; Yamin, 2009).

Research in psychiatric settings indicates that dignity is both an intrinsic, self-related process and a reciprocal, extrinsic/interpersonal experience. For instance, an individual's sense of dignity can be thwarted by positive and negative symptoms of SMI, specifically when these symptoms are misunderstood by others. On the other hand, dignity can be enhanced if the patient and significant others embrace a recovery-focused relationship in which they perceive themselves to be treated as an individual, thus reducing the shame that may be associated with being mentally ill (Skorpen et al., 2015). Being seen as human being who are equal, experiencing dignity despite the disease and frequent marginalization, and fighting for their own dignity are priorities for people with SMI.

6.3   Palliative Care in People with SMI

The existence of disparities in health and healthcare between patients with schizophrenia and/or SMI and patients without a diagnosis of mental illness is extremely important, especially, but not only in end-of-life care. A series of studies have shown that the problems of stigma are related to both social factors, such as poverty, lack of family support, and social isolation, as well as patient-level factors, such as cognitive impairment, psychiatric disabilities, and chronicity, all of which are implicated in the risk for poor end-of-life care among patients with SMI (Grassi & Riba, 2020; Riley et al., 2022; Sheridan, 2019).

In one of the first studies conducted in a palliative care setting, Chochinov et al. (2012) found that compared to their matched cohort, Canadian patients with schizophrenia were less likely to see specialists other than psychiatrists, less likely to be prescribed analgesics, and less likely to receive palliative care. They also were much more likely to die in nursing homes where physical, psychological, and spiritual care is possibly less optimal than in palliative care units (Martens et al., 2013). In a further Australian study (Spilsbury et al., 2018), patients with schizophrenia in the last year of life were less likely to be admitted to hospital and to have access to community-based specialty palliative care, but more likely to attend emergency departments. In general, what emerges is that stigma affects: quality of care and access to care; issues related to consent, the patient's capacity for their end-of-life care decisions, and the appointment of substitute decision makers; the practices of psychosocial interventions, pharmacology, family and healthcare collaborations, goals of care; communication, provider education, and access to care (Relyea et al., 2019). These data were more recently confirmed by other studies in Taiwan (Huang et al., 2018) and France (Fond et al., 2019). The latter was carried out on 2481 patients with schizophrenia and 9896 matched controls. The authors found that patients with schizophrenia were more likely to receive palliative care in the last 31 days of life and less likely to receive high-intensity end-of-life care (e.g., chemotherapy and surgery), were more likely to die younger, and had a shorter duration between cancer diagnosis and death than controls. More recently, a Swedish study, comparing 320 patients with psychosis with 24,056 patients without mental health problems, all at the end of life, found that the former group had a lower probability of receiving proper palliative care (Bergqvist et al., 2024).

6.4   Mechanisms Involved in Non-dignified End-of-Life Care Among People with SMI

When examining the reasons and causes of the inequalities identified above, several issues emerge (Shalev et al., 2020; McNamara et al., 2018). One issue regards the complications of information processing and communication determined by cognitive impairment and lack of insight that might derive from SMI. A second issue has to do with the problem of identifying caregivers in the home environment because of previous family disruption, sharing a house, living alone, or being homeless. A third aspect is about common concerns related to the assumption that the patient will be unmanageable, because of the lack of identifiable institutional or community care staff to provide adequate care or sufficient resources. Lastly, healthcare professionals report perceiving themselves as not sufficiently trained, holding wrong assumptions about SMI, lacking adequate educational resources, services, policies or guidelines, and experiencing fear and concernes about mental illness. These findings have been confirmed by a further qualitative study among palliative care nurses, who indicated six main themes as obstacles to dealing with patients with SMI:

stigma of mental illness, effect of SMI symptoms on communication and trust, chaotic family systems, advocacy issues around pain and comfort, need for formal support, no right place to die (Morgan, 2016).

In the context of cancer care, Irwin et al. (2014) have further indicated that interrelated patient-based, provider-based, and systems-based factors, influenced by mental health stigma, may impact not only cancer prevention, diagnosis, and treatment, but also end-of-life care. More specifically, the authors consider that disparities in cancer care for patients with schizophrenia (but it can be extended to other SMI) derive from several factors. On one side, patient inappropriate affect, positive or negative psychotic symptoms, cognitive symptoms (e.g., impaired attention and executive function), disorganized behaviour, dysfunctional coping (e.g., pathological denial), and poor health behaviours (e.g., poor adherence to treatment) contribute to the problem. On the other side, healthcare providers (e.g., GPs, oncologists, nurses) experience difficulties when they relate to people with these symptoms and with poor functioning, because the patient behaviour is often unfamiliar and incomprehensible to the clinical team. Fear of violent behaviour or suicide risk, and prejudice about the un-treatability of psychiatric conditions are further barriers for trust and proper care of patients with SMI. Finally, the fragmentation of healthcare services, the difficulty in creating a whole-person-centred approach, and the tendency of psychiatry and somatic medicine to work in a separate or non-integrated way are a third cause of the problem, which has been since many years described as a "scandal" in mental health settings (Thornicroft, 2011).

6.5   CONTRASTING INIQUITY AND INJUSTICE WITH PERSON-CENTRED AND DIGNITY-ORIENTED PSYCHIATRY

In order to contrast stigma and non-dignity-care for people with SMI, the Institutional Program on Psychiatry for the Person (IPPP) established by the 2005 General Assembly of the World Psychiatric Association (WPA), launched the initiative affirming the need for psychiatry to apply a model based on a whole-person approach. The articulation of science and humanism is the main framework used to gather all the relevant facts pertaining to the whole person. With respect to this, Person–Centred Psychiatry is more than the individualization of care or respect for patients' rights. It includes recognizing the individual subjectivity of the patient's whole person beyond the limits determined by the illness and its symptoms, therefore, using a dignity-oriented approach. The purpose of Person–Centred Psychiatry (Mezzich et al., 2016) is to promote care *of the person* (i.e., by pursuing the totality of the person's health), *for the person* (i.e., by promoting the fulfilment of the person's life projects), *by the person* (i.e., with clinicians extending themselves as full human beings with high ethical standards), and *with the person* (i.e., working in a collaborative and empowering manner with respect for each other) (Christodoulou et al., 2008; Mezzich, 2007). In a word, all these are attitudes and behaviours that ultimately reinforce dignity against stigma, marginalization, and epistemic injustice.

These principles are quite obvious, but are never underscored enough in clinical settings, including palliative care, as underlined elsewhere (Grassi et al., 2016). There is an urgent need for increased awareness of potential healthcare disparities, creative approaches in multidisciplinary care, and provision of adequate palliative services and resources that can enhance end-of-life care in schizophrenia (Baruth et al., 2021). There are four guiding principles of biomedical ethics to be followed in palliative care for people with SMI: (i) autonomy in relation to issues regarding the *decision-making capacity*; (ii) justice in relation to *access to quality care* to reduce the presence of stigma; and (iii) *non-maleficence* and (iv) *beneficence* in relation to the ongoing debate regarding the benefits and obstacles in applying palliative care in the context of psychiatry (Moureau et al., 2023). Personal virtues and attitudes in healthcare professionals, like compassion, non-abandonment, and upholding dignity of the patients, are key factors for implementing palliative care among this fragile segment of the population.

For these reasons, it is pivotal to improve education and training, including communication skills and assessment and management of emotions and psychiatric symptoms when dealing with people with SMI in order to increase the quality of their care (Cunningham et al., 2013). Hinrichs et al. (2022) consider some principles that should be basically applied in palliative care settings, although it is a challenging context, namely eliciting core care values and lending additional support to teams, via a fruitful interdisciplinary approach that enables to meet all the care needs of patients with life-limiting illness with the aim to achieve the best possible quality of life.

It is also paramount to actively find the most important person or carer (e.g., psychiatric case manager, nurse) in the patient's life to receive help in understanding what life-limiting illness means to that unique patient with the aim to offer value-based recommendations and treatment. What is applied in psychiatry by the recovery-based approach (Table 6.1) should be also taught to palliative care professionals, as a guide to deliver the best possible care at the end of life. The needs of each patient should be carefully monitored exploring the multiple issues related to individual representation of the illness, coping, and death and dying (Table 6.2), as emerged in a qualitative study of patients with SMI with terminal somatic diseases (Baruth et al., 2021; Knippenberg et al., 2023).

A series of recommendations have been underlined to improve the quality of palliative care among people with SMI (Callaway et al., 2021; Donald & Stajduhar, 2019; Woods et al., 2008), such as:

1. palliative care must be centred on the needs of the person with a therapeutic relationship based on respect, dignity, hope, and non-abandonment;
2. people with SMI have palliative care needs to be addressed as for all people, such as adequate pain and symptom control, maintenance of function, enhancement of quality of life, support for relationships, and possibility of dying with dignity;
3. need for service integration and continuity of care, interdisciplinary and interspecialty teamwork, communication, and outreach into community agencies and shelters;
4. cross-training in palliative care and mental health, integrating principles of hospice palliative care in end-of-life care for people with SMI in both palliative care and mental health settings.

If increasing dignity is one of the aims of palliative care for patients with SMI, specific treatment has been also developed for these purposes. With respect to this, Dignity Therapy (DT) is one of the possible interventions to enhance quality of life and to reduce the risk of negative consequences caused by stigma and epistemic injustice in palliative care (Russo, 2023). Developed by Chochinov (2012), DT is a brief, personalized, and empirically based intervention for patients with life-threatening or limiting illnesses. It aims to have patients talk about things that matter most to them, creating a permanent legacy that helps them strengthen

Table 6.1 Recovery-oriented strategy for palliative care settings (based on Hinrichs et al., 2022)

- Focus on preserving dignity
- Helping care team maintain empathy
- Highlighting an individual's unique strengths, abilities, and needs
- Acknowledging psychosocial complexities present in SMI
- Attempting to eradicate stigma around SMI
- Fostering control through shared decision-making
- Maintaining a core collaboration and open-mindedness

Table 6.2 Topics to be explored in palliative care for people with SMI (based on Hinrichs et al., 2022)

Beginning of the illness
- First symptoms
- First contact with a medical professional
- (Medical) treatment, care, and support
- Changes in social contact, work, and residency
- Current treatment, care, and support

Other symptoms or diseases
- Diseases and symptoms
- First contact with a medical professional
- (Medical) treatment, care, and support
- Changes in social contact, work, and residency
- Current treatment, care, and support

Further information about current treatment, care, and support
- Place of treatment
- Involved disciplines ➔ Tasks of involved disciplines
- Opinion about the treatment ➔ Example(s) and explanation of positive and negative experiences
- Improvement suggestions

Perception of the fact that the illness is incurable
- Patient's end of life ➔ Meaning, Involvement of others, Subjects discussed with others
- Expectations about final stage ➔ Treatment and support, Involved disciplines
- Experiences with end-of-life care so far ➔ Positive and negative experiences
- Needs and wishes

Current situation (Perceptions of health and health issues; Coping with illness and symptoms; Experiences with and wishes for current healthcare; Contact with relatives and coresidents; Experiences with the end of life of relatives and coresidents)

Anticipation of end of life (Willingness to discuss end of life and death; Wishes and expectations regarding one's own end of life; Practical aspects relating to matters after the death dignity and face their suffering. The protocol consists of 2–3 individual meetings within which the patient is firstly shown the DT questions and asked to consider what they might wish to speak about during the session. DT offers the participant an opportunity to reflect upon crucial existential and relational issues, and to review aspects of their lives and of self that they wish to be remembered.

This process focuses on tasks such as settling relationships, sharing words of love and wisdom with significant others, and preparing a legacy of memories and shared values. About a week later, the DT meeting is carried out and audio recorded. These meaningful memories, values, words of wisdom, and special messages are transcribed verbatim and then shaped into a narrative through a preliminary editing process. A session is dedicated to the final editing process with the participant, following which they are provided the final written a legacy (generativity) document, to be shared and passed along to family members and beloved ones. The ultimate intent of DT is to lessen distress, promote quality of life, validate personhood, alleviate suffering, and give meaning and purpose to life.

There are few experiences of applying the DT to the psychiatry settings (namely, three case reports of patients with depression, schizoaffective disorder; and a randomized clinical trial in patients with major depression) (Avery & Baez, 2012; Avery & Savitz, 2011; Julião, 2019; Solomita & Franza, 2022). DT appeared to increase the sense of hope in patients and to have a role in the patients regaining the sense that life is meaningful. In the only qualitative DT study intervention comparing patients with SMI (mainly schizophrenia and bipolar disorders) and patients with cancer, similar themes emerged within the generativity documents (Grassi et al., 2022). In fact, analysis of DT narratives among both groups of patients yielded similar categories, namely "Meaning" (theme examples "vitality", "self-evaluation", "pride", "evolution of self", "support"), "Resources" (theme examples "support", "resilience", "family", "encounters"), "Legacy" ("bequest for others", "time to say"), and "Dignity", as well as "Stigma". In this sense, the meaning of dignity for patients with SMI was related to the values that are an integral part of the dignity model, specifically self-worth and self-esteem, autonomy and control, purpose, identity and continuity, relatedness and connectedness, love, and comfort.

Although DT has not yet applied to patients with SMI in the setting of palliative care, these preliminary results seem to be in line with the results of many studies using DT in patients without SMI at the end of life, as shown by recent reviews and metanalyses (Cuevas et al., 2021; Gagnon Mailhot et al., 2022; Li et al., 2020; Martínez et al., 2017; Zhang et al., 2022).

The person-centred approach and treatment of patients in advanced phases of illness, and at the end of life is a basic requirement for multidisciplinary teams in medicine. This is mandatory for patients affected by SMI, who have the right to receive optimal palliative care, based on compassion, empathy, responsiveness to needs, values, and expressed preferences; emotional support, relief of fear and anxiety; physical comfort, as part of any healthcare professional armamentarium in the relationship with the patient (Kissane, 2000). This can facilitate the possibility for individuals to express their representation of illness, giving to the narrative dimension of their experience, the sense of epistemic justice, as underscored above (Hultman & Hultman, 2023; Mooney et al., 2023).

In order to reduce the alienation of those affected by mental illness, person-centred psychiatry promotes a medicine of the person, for the person, by the person, and with the person. Dignity-conserving care is part of this approach and it should be practised in mental healthcare settings, enabling partnerships with people encountering psychiatric disorders that include mitigating loss of identity, shattering of their self-image, and various challenges within the psychological, interpersonal, spiritual, and existential domains. All these aspects are further posed at end of life, with needs that should be mandatorily addressed, such as: finding hope and meaning in life, finding spiritual resources, having someone to talk to, finding peace of mind, help in solving concerns, support in dealing with possible feelings of guilt, worthlessness, disvalue of not having made a meaningful and/or lasting contribution in one's own life. In this sense, dignity-conserving care represents a framework to increase epistemic justice involved in that individual person, irrespective of their physical (i.e., advanced stage of illness and end of life) or psychological/psychopathological condition (i.e., SMI).

Acknowledgements Luigi Grassi and Martino Belvederi Murri are grateful for the support of project EPIC (Epistemic Injustice in Healthcare, 2023–2029), generously funded by a Wellcome Discovery Award and led by Havi Carel at the University of Bristol. The work has been also supported by: #NEXTGENERATIONEU (NGEU) project MNESYS (PE0000006)—A Multiscale integrated approach to the study of the nervous system in health and disease (DN. 1553 11.10.2022) funded by the Ministry of University and Research (MUR),

National Recovery and Resilience Plan (NRRP); #NEXTGENERATIONEU (NGEU) project PNRR-MAD-2022-12375899 "Cost-effectiveness of innovative, non-pharmacological strategies for early detection, prevention and tailored care of depressive disorders among cancer patients: Transcranial Magnetic Stimulation and Virtual Reality based Cognitive Remediation", funded by the Ministry of Health, National Recovery and Resilience Plan (NRRP).

REFERENCES

Alcalde, J., & Zimmermann, C. (2022, April 28). Stigma about palliative care: Origins and solutions. *Ecancermedicalscience, 16*, 1377. https://doi.org/10.3332/ecancer.2022.1377

Avery, J. D., & Baez, M. A. (2012). Dignity therapy for major depressive disorder: A case report. *Journal of Palliative Medicine, 15*, 509–509.

Avery, J. D., & Savitz, A. J. (2011). A novel use of dignity therapy. *American Journal of Psychiatry, 168*, 1340–1340.

Barclay, L. (2016). In sickness and in dignity: A philosophical account of the meaning of dignity in health care. *International Journal of Nursing Studies, 61*, 136–141.

Baruth, J. M., Ho, J. B., Mohammad, S. I., & Lapid, M. I. (2021, February). End-of-life care in schizophrenia: A systematic review. *International Psychogeriatrics, 33*(2), 129–147.

Bergqvist, J., Hedskog, S., Hedman, C., Schultz, T., & Strang, P. (2024, April). Patients with both cancer and psychosis-to what extent do they receive specialized palliative care. *Acta Psychiatrica Scandinavica, 149*(4), 313–322.

Bhugra, D., Ventriglio, A., & Pathare, S. (2016). Freedom and equality in dignity and rights for persons with mental illness. *The Lancet. Psychiatry, 3*(3), 196–197.

Burns, J. K. (2009). Mental health and inequity: A human rights approach to inequality, discrimination, and mental disability. *Health and Human Rights, 11*(2), 19–31.

Callaway, C. A., Corveleyn, A. E., Barry, M. J., Gorton, E. I., Nierenberg, A. A., & Irwin, K. E. (2021, December). Lessons learned: Building a coalition to advance equity in cancer and mental health care. *Psychooncology, 30*(12), 2087–2091.

Chochinov, H. M. (2002). Dignity-conserving care—A new model for palliative care: Helping the patient feel valued. *JAMA, 287*(17), 2253–2260.

Chochinov, H. M. (2006). Dignity in care: A definition and framework for assessment. *Journal of Palliative Medicine, 9*(2), 297–303.

Chochinov, H. M. (2012). *Dignity therapy: A patient-centered approach for improving end-of-life care.* Oxford University Press.

Chochinov, H. M., Hack, T., McClement, S., Kristjanson, L., & Harlos, M. (2002). Dignity in the terminally ill: A developing empirical model. *Social Science & Medicine, 54,* 433–443.

Chochinov, H. M., Martens, P. J., Prior, H. J., & Kredentser, M. S. (2012). Comparative health care use patterns of people with schizophrenia near the end of life: A population-based study in Manitoba, Canada. *Schizophrenia Research, 141,* 241–246.

Christodoulou, G., Fulford, B., & Mezzich, J. E. (2008). Psychiatry for the person and its conceptual bases. *International Psychiatry: Bulletin of the Board of International Affairs of the Royal College of Psychiatrists, 5*(1), 1–3.

Corrigan, P. W., & Watson, A. C. (2002). Understanding the impact of stigma on people with mental illness. *World Psychiatry: Official Journal of the World Psychiatric Association (WPA), 1*(1), 16–20.

Corrigan, P. W., Watson, A. C., & Ottati, V. (2003). From whence comes mental illness stigma? *The International Journal of Social Psychiatry, 49*(2), 142–157.

Cuevas, P. E., Davidson, P., Mejilla, J., & Rodney, T. (2021, February 25). Dignity therapy for end-of-life care patients: A literature review. *Journal of Patient Experience, 8,* 2374373521996951.

Cunningham, C., Peters, K., & Mannix, J. (2013). Physical health inequities in people with severe mental illness: Identifying initiatives for practice change. *Issues in Mental Health Nursing, 34*(12), 855–862.

Donald, E. E., & Stajduhar, K. I. (2019, August). A scoping review of palliative care for persons with severe persistent mental illness. *Palliat Support Care, 17*(4), 479–487.

Drożdżowicz, A. (2021, February 19). Epistemic injustice in psychiatric practice: Epistemic duties and the phenomenological approach. *Journal of Medical Ethics.* https://doi.org/10.1136/medethics-2020-106679

Fond, G., Salas, S., Pauly, V., Baumstarck, K., Bernard, C., Orleans, V., Llorca, P. M., Lancon, C., Auquier, P., & Boyer, L. (2019). End-of-life care among patients with schizophrenia and cancer: A population-based cohort study from the French national hospital database. *Lancet Public Health, 4*(11), e583–e591.

Formagini, T., Poague, C., O'Neal, A., & Brooks, J. V. (2022, January). "When I heard the word palliative": Obscuring and clarifying factors affecting the stigma around palliative care referral in oncology. *JCO Oncology Practice, 18*(1), e72–e79. https://doi.org/10.1200/OP.21.00088

Fricker, M. (2007). *Epistemic injustice: Power and the ethics of knowing.* Oxford University Press.

Gagnon Mailhot, M., Léonard, G., Gadoury-Sansfaçon, G.-P., Stout, D., & Ellefsen, É. (2022). A scoping review on the experience of participating in dignity therapy for adults at the end of life. *Journal of Palliative Medicine, 25,* 1143–1150.

Grassi, L. (manuscript in preparation). Stigma and dignity as two faces of the same coin in psychiatry.

Grassi, L., & Chochinov, H. M. (2024). Beyond the limits of mental illness: Dignity and dignity therapy in person-centered psychiatry. In I. Testoni, F. Scardigli, & A. Toniolo (Eds.), *Eternity between space and time: From consciousness to the cosmos* (pp. 257–270). Walter de Gruyter.

Grassi, L., Chochinov, H., Moretto, G., & Nanni, M. (2019). Dignity-conserving care in medicine. In G. L. In, M. Riba, & T. Wise (Eds.), *Person centered approach to recovery in medicine* (pp. 97–115). Springer.

Grassi, L., Nanni, M. G., Caruso, R., et al. (2022). A comparison of dignity therapy narratives among people with severe mental illness and people with cancer. *Psycho-Oncology, 31*, 676–679.

Grassi, L., Nanni, M. G., Riba, M. B., & Folesani, F. (2024, June). Dignity in medicine: Definition, assessment and therapy. *Current Psychiatry Reports, 26*(6), 273–293. https://doi.org/10.1007/s11920-024-01506-3

Grassi, L., & Riba, M. (2020, October). Cancer and severe mental illness: Bi-directional problems and potential solutions. *Psychooncology, 29*(10), 1445–1451.

Grassi, L., Riba, M., Bras, M., & Glare, P. (2016). Person-centered palliative care. In J. E. Mezzich, M. Botbol, G. N. Christodoulou, C. R. Cloninger, & I. M. Salloum (Eds.), *Person centered psychiatry* (pp. 487–500). Springer/ Springer Nature. https://doi.org/10.1007/978-3-319-39724-5_35

Grassi, L., Riba, M., McFarland, D., Ferrara, M., Zaffarani, G., Cruciata, M., & Caruso, R. (in press) The challenging problem of cancer care in patients with Sever Mental Illness (SMI). *Current Psychiatry Reports*.

Gray, A. J. (2002, February). Stigma in psychiatry. *Journal of the Royal Society of Medicine, 95*(2), 72–76.

Hassall, R. (2024). Sense-making and hermeneutical injustice following a psychiatric diagnosis. *Journal of Evaluation in Clinical Practice*. https://doi.org/ 10.1111/jep.13971

Hinrichs, K. L. M., Woolverton, C. B., & Meyerson, J. L. (2022, February). Help me understand: Providing palliative care to individuals with serious mental illness. *American Journal of Hospice and Palliative Medicine Care, 39*(2), 250–257.

Hinshaw, S., & Stier, A. (2008). Stigma as related to mental disorders. *Annual Review of Clinical Psychology, 4*, 367–393.

Huang, H. K., Wang, Y. W., Hsieh, J. G., & Hsieh, C. J. (2018, May). Disparity of end-of-life care in cancer patients with and without schizophrenia: A nationwide population-based cohort study. *Schizophrenia Research, 195*, 434–440.

Hultman, L., & Hultman, M. (2023). "Believe me, only I know how I feel." An autoethnographic account of experiences of epistemic injustice in mental health care. *Frontiers in Psychiatry, 14*, 1058422. https://doi.org/10.3389/fpsyt.2023.1058422

Irwin, K. E., Henderson, D. C., Knight, H. P., & Pirl, W. F. (2014). Cancer care for individuals with schizophrenia. *Cancer, 120*(3), 323–334.

Jacobson, N. (2007). Dignity and health: A review. *Social Science & Medicine, 64*, 292–302.

Julião, M. (2019, January–February). The use of dignity therapy beyond terminal illness: A case report. *Psychosomatics, 60*(1), 101.

Kissane, D. W. (2000). Psychospiritual and existential distress. The challenge for palliative care. *Australian Family Physician, 29*(11), 1022–1025.

Knippenberg, I., Zaghouli, N., Engels, Y., Vissers, K. C. P., & Groot, M. M. (2023, September). Severe mental illness and palliative care: Patient semistructured interviews. *BMJ Supportive and Palliative Care, 13*(3), 331–337.

Lawrence, D., & Kisely, S. (2010). Inequalities in healthcare provision for people with severe mental illness. *Journal of Psychopharmacology, 24*(4 Suppl.), 61–68.

Lebech, M. (2009). *On the problem of human dignity. A hermenutical and phenomenolgical investigation*. Königshausen & Neumann.

Li, Y., Li, X., Hou, L., Cao, L., Liu, G., & Yang, K. (2020). Effectiveness of dignity therapy for patients with advanced cancer: A systematic review and meta-analysis of 10 randomized controlled trials. *Depression and Anxiety, 37*, 234–246.

Livingston, J. D., & Boyd, J. E. (2010). Correlates and consequences of internalized stigma for people living with mental illness: A systematic review and meta-analysis. *Social Science & Medicine, 71*(12), 2150–2161. https://doi.org/10.1016/j.socscimed.2010.09.030

Macklin, R. (2003, December 20). Dignity is a useless concept. *BMJ, 327*(7429), 1419–1420.

Martens, P. J., Chochinov, H. M., & Prior, H. J. (2013). Where and how people with schizophrenia die: A population-based, matched-cohort study in Manitoba, Canada. *Journal of Clinical Psychiatry, 74*, e551–e557.

Martínez, M., Arantzamendi, M., Belar, A., Carrasco, J. M., Carvajal, A., Rullán, M., & Centeno, C. (2017). 'Dignity therapy', a promising intervention in palliative care: A comprehensive systematic literature review. *Palliative Medicine, 31*, 492–509.

McNamara, B., Same, A., Rosenwax, L., & Kelly, B. (2018). Palliative care for people with schizophrenia: A qualitative study of an under-serviced group in need. *BMC Palliative Care, 17*, 53.

Mestdagh, A., & Hansen, B. (2014). Stigma in patients with schizophrenia receiving community mental health care: A review of qualitative studies. *Social Psychiatry and Psychiatric Epidemiology, 49*(1), 79–87. https://doi.org/10.1007/s00127-013-0729-4

Mezzich, J. E. (2007). Psychiatry for the person: Articulating medicine's science and humanism. *World Psychiatry, 6*(2), 65–67.

Mezzich, J. E., Botbol, M., Christodoulou, G. N., Cloninger, C. R., & Salloum, I. M. (Eds.). (2016). *Person centered psychiatry*. Springer.

Mooney, R., Dempsey, C., Brown, B. J., Keating, F., Joseph, D., & Bhui, K. (2023). Using participatory action research methods to address epistemic injustice within mental health research and the mental health system. *Frontiers in Public Health, 11*, 1075363. https://doi.org/10.3389/fpubh.2023.1075363

Morgan, B. D. (2016, January–February). "No right place to die": Nursing attitudes and needs in caring for people with serious mental illness at end-of-life. *Journal of the American Psychiatric Nurses Association, 22*(1), 31–34.

Moureau, L., Verhofstadt, M., & Liégeois, A. (2023, March). Mapping the ethical aspects in end-of-life care for persons with a severe and persistent mental illness: A scoping review of the literature. *Front Psychiatry, 16*(14), 1094038.

Pellegrino, E. (2008). The lived experience of human dignity. In *Human dignity and bioethics* (pp. 513–540). Essays commissioned by the President's Council of Bioethics.

Relyea, E., MacDonald, B., Cattaruzza, C., & Marshall, D. (2019). On the margins of death: A scoping review on palliative care and schizophrenia. *Journal of Palliative Care, 34*(1), 62–69.

Riley, K., Hupcey, J. E., & Kowalchik, K. J. (2022, June 1). Palliative care in severe and persistent mental illness: A systematic review. *Journal of Hospice and Palliative Nursing, 24*(3), E88–E93.

Ritunnano, R. (2022). Overcoming hermeneutical injustice in mental health: A role for critical phenomenology. *Journal of the British Society for Phenomenology, 53*, 243–260.

Rosen, M. (2012). *Dignity. Its history and meaning*. Harvard University Press.

Russo, J. (2023). Psychiatrization, assertions of epistemic justice, and the question of agency. *Frontiers in Sociology, 8*, 1092298. https://doi.org/10.3389/fsoc.2023.1092298

Sakakibara, E. (2023). Epistemic injustice in the therapeutic relationship in psychiatry. *Theoretical Medicine and Bioethics, 44*(5), 477–502. https://doi.org/10.1007/s11017-023-09627-1

Shalev, D., Fields, L., & Shapiro, P. A. (2020, September–October). End-of-life care in individuals with serious mental illness. *Psychosomatics, 61*(5), 428–435.

Shen, M. J., & Wellman, J. D. (2019, August). Evidence of palliative care stigma: The role of negative stereotypes in preventing willingness to use palliative care. *Palliative and Support Care, 17*(4), 374–380. https://doi.org/10.1017/S1478951518000834

Sheridan, A. J. (2019, November). Palliative care for people with serious mental illnesses. *Lancet Public Health, 4*(11), e545–e546.

Skorpen, F., Rehnsfeldt, A., & Thorsen, A. A. (2015). The significance of small things for dignity in psychiatric care. *Nursing Ethics, 22*(7), 754–764.

Skorpen, F., Thorsen, A. A., Forsberg, C., & Rehnsfeldt, A. W. (2014). Suffering related to dignity among patients at a psychiatric hospital. *Nursing Ethics, 21*(2), 148–162.

Slack, S. K., & Barclay, L. (2023). First-person disavowals of digital phenotyping and epistemic injustice in psychiatry. *Medicine, Health Care and Philosophy, 26*(4), 605–614. https://doi.org/10.1007/s11019-023-10174-8

Solomita, B., & Franza, F. (2022, September). Dignity-therapy in bipolar disorder and major depression: An observational study in a psychiatric rehabilitation center. *Psychiatria Danubina, 34*(Suppl. 8), 71–74.

Spencer, L. (2023). Hermeneutical injustice and unworlding in psychopathology. *Philosophical Psychology, 36*(7), 1300–1325. https://doi.org/10.1080/095 15089.2023.2166821

Spiegelberg, H. (1971). Human dignity: A challenge to contemporary philosophy. *The Philosophy Forum, 9*, 39–64.

Spilsbury, K., Rosenwax, L., Brameld, K., Kelly, B., & Arendts, G. (2018). Morbidity burden and community-based palliative care are associated with rates of hospital use by people with schizophrenia in the last year of life: A population-based matched cohort study. *PLoS ONE, 13*(11), e0208220.

Thornicroft, G. (2011). Physical health disparities and mental illness: The scandal of premature mortality. *British Journal of Psychiatry, 199*(6), 441–442.

Whitley, R., & Campbell, R. D. (2014). Stigma, agency and recovery amongst people with severe mental illness. *Social Science and Medicine, 107*, 1–8.

WHO Mental Health Action Plan 2013–2030. www.who.int/publications/i/item/9789240031029

Woods, A., Willison, K., Kington, C., & Gavin, A. (2008, November). Palliative care for people with severe persistent mental illness: A review of the literature. *Canadian Journal of Psychiatry, 53*(11), 725–736.

Xiao, J., Ng, M. S. N., Yan, T., Chow, K. M., & Chan, C. W. H. (2021). How patients with cancer experience dignity: An integrative review. *Psycho-Oncology, 30*, 1220–1231.

Yamin, A. E. (2009). Shades of dignity: Exploring the demands of equality in applying human rights frameworks to health. *Health and Human Rights, 11*(2), 1–18.

Zhang, Y., Li, J., & Hu, X. (2022, August). The effectiveness of dignity therapy on hope, quality of life, anxiety, and depression in cancer patients: A meta-analysis of randomized controlled trials. *International Journal of Nursing Studies, 132*, 104273.

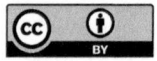

CHAPTER 7

Promoting Good Living and Social Health in Dementia

Rabih Chattat⊚, Sara Trolese⊚, and Ilaria Chirico⊚

Abstract The notion of good living in chronic disease in general and, in the case of dementia specifically, highlights the role of social health in preserving the well-being of the people involved. In ageing ageism, discrimination toward older adults is considered an important barrier against involvement in society. In the case of dementia, stigmatisation can have an impact on the person affected, on the family, on healthcare services, and on society more widely. Examples of the impact of discrimination are related to diagnosis disclosure, advance care planning, and the involvement of people with dementia in decision-making about their future treatment. Furthermore, the labelling of the behaviour of people with dementia as a disorder is a way to pathologise it and does not take into account the role of relationships and the social context as a drive for the behaviour itself. As a result of the stigmatisation and the labelling, people with dementia experience epistemic injustice as they are considered neither partners in the decision-making process nor full members of

R. Chattat (✉) · S. Trolese · I. Chirico
Department of Psychology, University of Bologna, Bologna, Italy
e-mail: rabih.chattat@unibo.it

© The Author(s) 2025
L. Bortolotti (ed.), *Epistemic Justice in Mental Healthcare*,
https://doi.org/10.1007/978-3-031-68881-2_7

125

society. A capability-based approach is needed to promote good living and social participation in people with dementia.

Keywords Dementia · Stigma · Social inclusion · Ageism · Well-being

7.1   HEALTH AND AGE-RELATED DISCRIMINATION

Chronic diseases impose a burden at a global level. The increase in life expectancy led to a growing number of older people with chronic health conditions such as cardiovascular disease, cancer, and neurodegenerative disease. Huber and colleagues (2011) highlighted the need to reconsider the definition of health as "the ability to adapt and to self-manage, in the face of social, physical and emotional challenges", rather than merely the presence or absence of a disease. The authors propose three domains of health: physical, psychological, and social health. Within this conceptualization, social health includes, from an individual perspective, three dimensions: (1) the capacity to fulfil potential and obligation; (2) the ability to manage life with some independence despite medical conditions; and (3) the ability to participate in social activities including work.

Beyond the individual level, a social-environmental level has been proposed (Vernooij-Dassen et al., 2022) which includes three different domains related to the structure (in terms of the type of social interaction such as social network size and composition, marital status, and frequency of contact), the function (such as emotional support and instrumental aids), and appraisal of the quality of relationships and interactions (related to the perception and interpretation of social contacts and consequent loneliness). Using the individual and social perspective, the authors argued that the individuals' functioning does not depend on their capacities only. The behaviour of their social environment which may support but also hinder them from using their capacities may be equally important. Social factors can influence older adults' psychological well-being and cognitive functioning, and they can enhance their cognitive reserve as well as they can moderate the progression of their cognitive decline (Samtani et al., 2022; Seifert et al., 2022). From this perspective, promoting social health and reducing isolation and discrimination can be considered as a treatment opportunity.

The role and importance of social aspects in promoting older adults' well-being and adaptation have been also discussed within the framework of age-related stigma and discrimination. A large body of literature outlined the role of stigma and discrimination toward ageing, frailty, and mental disease. Terms such as "ageism" (i.e., discrimination toward older adults), which was first proposed by Butler (1969), are used today to describe any kind of stereotype, prejudice, and discrimination toward a social group based on chronological age. It can be directed toward adolescents and older adults mainly by adults. Ageism toward older adults is now recognised as an important issue to be addressed to promote healthy Ageing. The United Nations General Assembly in their plan for the decade (2021–2030) of Healthy aging suggested, as a first action, to combat ageism. Stigma toward ageing is related to "how we think, feel and act towards age and ageing" focusing the attention on the role of the social context and the role of others and on how norms, policies, attitudes, and approaches can exclude people from access to facilities, services, and resources.

The stigmatisation of older adults in general, and of those with chronic illness specifically, can have a significant impact on health and well-being (Kang & Kim, 2022), thus implying stereotype internalisation by older adults through self-stigmatisation, isolation, and loneliness. The consequences of ageism and "self-ageism" also impact the access to care, and the quality of care for older people in different settings.

As mentioned before, stigmatisation of older people is even more important in the case of a chronic illness and, specifically, in the domain of mental health. The attitudes of mental health professionals toward psychological interventions with older people are influenced by negative ideas regarding the ability of older people to benefit from such treatments (Bodner, 2009). For example, in many countries, specific training for mental health professionals on the approach to mental disorders in older people is not available. Assessment criteria, pharmacological treatment, and psychotherapies are based on the work with adults and transferred to the work in geriatrics. Similarly, the research in these domains is lacking in addressing the specific conditions of older people.

Within mental health domains, neurodegenerative diseases, and mainly dementia, are considered a public health priority, looking at prevalence and incidence rates and the lack of a cure until now. The link between dementia and age is widely recognised and the prevalence of the disease increases with age, which is considered one of the most important risk factors for dementia. However, adults can also be affected by dementia, and this condition is called "young onset dementia". Since the prevalence of dementia is growing with age, people living with this condition can be exposed to a double type of stigma, one related to age (Ageism) and one related to dementia (demente-ism) (Brooker, 2007; Evans, 2018).

Dementia, a neurodegenerative disorder, is an umbrella term used to indicate a variety of conditions characterised by neuronal damage. The most prevalent type of dementia is Alzheimer's disease which accounts for around 62% of all types of dementia followed by vascular dementia, frontotemporal dementia, and Lewy body dementia as the most frequent. Dementia, a brain disease, is characterised by a progressive decline in several domains of cognitive abilities such as executive functions, learning and memory, language, perceptual and motor functions, complex attention, and social cognition (DSM-5). The duration is up to 12–15 years. Cognitive decline has an impact on the person's capacity to retain information and also to recall memories, communicate and understand others and the world around them, and to perform daily activities. The person becomes more and more dependent in managing daily life, thus relying on others to perform simple activities in the advanced stages of dementia. Another disease aspect, beyond cognitive and functional decline, is the presence of the so-called "behavioural and psychological symptoms" such as delusions, hallucinations, anxiety, depression, and agitation. These noncognitive symptoms represent a challenge for carers, impacting on the quality of life of people with dementia and their family caregivers as well representing the major cause of institutionalisation.

Dementia has long been considered as a biological disorder (Vernooij-Dassen et al., 2021) caused mainly by brain damage. The consequences of brain damage on cognitive abilities lead, as mentioned above, to people's difficulties in verbal communication (understanding and expression), in their capacity to cope with everyday challenges such as managing finances, preparing meals, dressing, or moving around. Several needs of people with dementia are unmet. Not only practical needs but also emotional and relational needs. Kitwood (1997) along with other authors (Sabat & Lee, 2012) are among the first researchers who propose the necessity to consider the person with dementia instead of dementia, thus highlighting the concepts of Personhood, and Selfhood.

Kitwood addressed the issue of malignant social psychology to describe how people with dementia are approached and treated by others. In his book, he used several terms to describe the approach of carers such as infantilization, intimidation, labelling by the name of the disease, invalidation, banishment, ignoring, mockery, and withholding.

All these terms outline the difficulty of professional carers to recognise and treat the person with dementia as a person, acting like it is not present in the interaction and the relationship. This way of approaching people with dementia has an impact on their experience of their condition. Many of the so-called "behavioural and psychological symptoms" of dementia can be considered as a reaction, a way to communicate, react or express unmet needs, or negative emotions related to the experience of the disease (Burley et al., 2021).

The work of Kitwood has been remarkable in the field of dementia care promoting a change in the understanding of the experience of people with dementia, and several actions have been undertaken to reduce stigma and social isolation. Nevertheless, the stigma toward people with dementia still needs to be addressed, since it has an impact on several aspects of the dementia journey from research to care and to social engagement.

7.2   STIGMA AND DEMENTIA: THE IMPACT

The impact of stigma toward dementia can be considered at different levels: the individual, the family, society, healthcare and welfare, research, and policies.

At an individual level, stigma can lead to feelings of shame, low self-esteem, a sense of uselessness, withdrawal from social interaction, social isolation, depression, and anxiety. People with dementia, challenged by the consequences of cognitive decline, experience several limitations which impact on their emotional balance.

Families are involved as well by experiencing feelings of shame, isolation, depression, and burden. Some authors suggest the term "courtesy stigma" or "associative stigma" to refer to the discrimination and prejudice experienced by people, because they are parents or relatives of a person with dementia (Van den Bossche & Scoenmakers, 2022). Another term proposed is the "affiliate stigma" to refer to the internalisation of the stigma by family caregivers with negative feelings toward themselves.

At the healthcare and welfare level, the stigmatisation of people with dementia can be observed at different stages across the care pathway. Since these aspects are related to the context, The multifaceted impact of stigmatisation in dementia will be discussed in detail.

At the societal level, the stigma of people with dementia can lead to the avoidance of contact and engagement, exclusion from social participation and involvement in social life, and the loss of friendships which in turn leads to social isolation and loneliness.

7.2.1   The Diagnosis Disclosure

Even if a lot of advances have been made for a timely diagnosis of dementia, a delay in diagnosis, which differs between countries across Europe and globally, is still observed, and it can last to 3–4 years from the onset of cognitive decline. Even after several public campaigns, the delay is still present and is related mainly to the reluctance of the person with dementia to seek help (37%), the lack of recognition by professionals of the signs of cognitive decline (33%), the attribution of cognitive changes to age (26%), and to the length of the diagnostic process (12%) (Woods et al., 2019). These results outline a combination of a lack of awareness by both professionals and people with cognitive problems and their reluctance to seek help, which is frequently associated with the fear of stigma.

The diagnosis disclosure is also another challenge in dementia care. Even if in most countries it is a right for people to receive information about their health condition and it is their own decision to share health information with others, in the case of dementia this right is not fully respected. In a survey collected in 5 European countries, several differences emerge. The direct communication of the diagnosis to the person with dementia ranges from 40% to 99%, and the lack of direct communication is partly is related to the expressed wishes of the person itself while, in large part, it is related to the decision of the healthcare professional or an explicit request of the family caregiver (Woods et al., 2019). In other studies, only 34% of primary care physicians communicate the diagnosis to the person with dementia (Low et al., 2019). Barriers to disclosing the diagnosis of dementia are at different levels (Wollney et al., 2022). At the clinician level, some reported barriers are related to the lack of training, the perceived lack of benefit in diagnosing dementia, the concern for the patient or the caregiver's response, and the capacity of the person with dementia to understand and retain information. At the patient/family level, the barriers are related to the lack of the ability to understand the diagnosis, and to the fears related to the disease. A systematic review (Yates et al., 2021) focused on the issue of diagnosis disclosure from the perspectives of healthcare professionals, carers, and people with dementia. The authors outline that research is needed to understand the perspectives of people with dementia regarding the process of diagnosis disclosure which can help the development of an approach which is reasonable for all actors involved in the process. In other words, there is a lack of research regarding how people with dementia experience the disclosure. It is difficult to disclose the diagnosis to a person with dementia and there is limited research on their experience within this process. Considering dementia as a process of decline, characterised by a loss of capacity, may lead to the person being excluded and losing their agency. Kate Swaffer (2015), a person with dementia, described "prescribed disengagement" (the post-diagnostic prescription to give up some of their usual activities) as increasing stigma and discrimination, reducing self-esteem, and devaluing and demeaning the person affected by this condition. This process of de-personalization leads to the exclusion of the person with dementia from being an agent, a person with rights in need to be heard by others. The consequences can have a significant impact on the person's good living and social health.

7.2.2 Advance Care Planning

In several dementia care pathways, the diagnosis disclosure should prepare for care planning or advanced care planning looking to the future of the person with dementia, where the loss of capacities may limit their chance to take part in some decisions about care.

In this domain, diagnostic disclosure plays an important role and only if people with dementia are aware of their conditions, a discussion about the future is feasible. We can mention two main barriers at this level. The first one is related to the attitude of professional carers who avoid talking about the prognosis of the disease. As for the diagnostic disclosure, prejudice about the capacity to understand and discuss care options is a limitation. Furthermore, the absence of a planned process for supporting people with dementia to accept and adapt to the new situation makes planning difficult. There are few structured approaches to follow-up the patient elaboration of the new information, which can support carers and people with dementia, and facilitate further discussion and a better way to deal with trauma-related to the loss of capacities and the planned future (Yates et al., 2021).

7.2.3   Shared Decision-Making

The post-diagnostic phase of dementia, which can last for several years, is usually divided into three stages that are mild, moderate, and severe (or advanced) dementia. The brain damage is more extended, and the loss of cognitive abilities is significant with consequences on the loss of autonomy and a greater dependency. Along the trajectory it is a great challenge to decide when the person with dementia loses their capacity to make decisions and also to establish what the content of the decision is. For example, at the mild-moderate stage, the person may be unable to understand a complex situation, but they are still capable of agreeing/ disagreeing with aspects related to daily life, such as participation in activities or comfortable/uncomfortable situations.

The most important barriers in long-term care toward shared decision-making and care planning for people with dementia are the attitudes of care professionals and family caregivers, the lack of professional training in communication skills as well as norms and job overload (Mariani et al., 2017). As in the diagnosis disclosure and advance care planning, the lack of involvement of people with dementia in decisions is related to the attitude of others toward the person with dementia and the non-recognition of their ability to communicate or express preferences and wishes. Even in the severe phase of dementia, the person is still able to react to external stimuli and express at least states of pleasure or pain, comfort, or discomfort. What is needed is a change in the way carers look at the person with dementia, recognising strengths along with limitations.

7.2.4   The So-Called Behavioral and Psychological Symptoms of Dementia (BPSD)

Kitwood (1997), writing about malignant social psychology, uses the term "labelling", which can be understood as naming a person by their disease or symptoms. In the domain of dementia, there is a group of symptoms labelled as behavioural and psychological symptoms of dementia (1996). This category includes aspects related to perceptions and thoughts (delusions, hallucinations and misperception), mood (anxiety, depression, apathy and emotional lability), behaviour (agitation, wandering, verbal and non-verbal behaviour which can be aggressive or not), sleep and eating changes. These features are considered as symptoms

of dementia related to brain damage, which means that they are meaning-
less and the main approach should consist of controlling and restraining
the person living with dementia. From the perspective of Person-centred
care (Kitwood, 1997) the behaviour can be considered as an expression
of unmet needs or as an expression of challenges or difficulties in coping
with changes related to cognitive limitations. Subsequently, Stokes (2000)
suggested the use of the term "challenging behaviour" to describe these
symptoms in order to understand the determinants of the behaviour, thus
underlining the need to find the meaning of certain behaviour in terms
of the needs, desires, and preferences of the person living with dementia.

In the NICE guidelines (2006), the term "behaviour that challenges"
has been used to outline that a certain behaviour can be seen as a reaction or a communication of the person regarding the experience of unmet
needs or distress or the absence of engagement. The main aim is to
cope with the changing situation and to maintain balance and well-being.
Recently, the NICE guidelines (2018) and the Italian guidelines for diagnosis and treatment of MCI and dementia use the term "non-cognitive
symptoms" of dementia, while other countries such as Canada or Australia
suggest others as well. What is important to consider is the effort needed
to reframe the concept and to shift from a "pathologizing" approach to
behaviour (Dupuis et al., 2012) toward an approach where the behaviour
is seen as a meaningful communication, and the challenge is related to
the capacity of carers to understand, underlying the determinants of the
behaviour and respond appropriately.

Burley et al. (2021) reported the perspectives of people with dementia
and their carers about BPSD. The results outlined the need for a
reframing of the concept for a better understanding of the experience of
the person with dementia. For example, the authors discussed that the use
of the term agitation can be misleading, while a better description such
as being frustrated or receiving discriminatory behaviour or inadequate
support can better represent the real experience faced by the person themselves. The debate around the issue of behaviour in dementia highlighted
the difficulty of carers in particular, but also of the public in general, to
recognise an active role of the person with dementia in the interaction
with the environment and others (carers, friends, and neighbours).

7.2.5   Behaviour Across the Trajectory of Dementia

As mentioned before, the progressive loss of cognitive abilities, specifically the capacity to use verbal communication, implies the use of non-verbal communication as a main skill to interact and exchange with others and the world. Motor activities (body language) as well as facial and vocal expressions become the most used tools to express and react to challenges faced by the person with dementia. Labelling these modalities as "symptoms of disease" implies denying the presence of the person, their history, their preferences and wishes, and their difficulties.

In this way, the process of objectivation (Kitwood, 1997) can lead to a complete absence of the other. The lack of awareness about the capacities and abilities of the person with dementia, even in the severe disease stage, undermines the inalienable human rights of the person.

7.3   Good Living with Dementia

The lack of a cure for dementia stimulates a large body of research aimed at promoting the well-being of people with dementia and their family caregivers. In recent years, there has been a global effort to refrain the vision of care for dementia from a "giving up" approach where, in the absence of treatment people are invited to "give up work, study, and to go home and live the time left" (Swaffer, 2015), to a more balanced approach where the focus is on good care and on promoting the quality of life and adaptation to the consequences of the disease. To achieve this objective, many researchers focus on interventions aimed at promoting psychological and social well-being. A large field has been developed regarding non-pharmacologic interventions or more specifically psychosocial interventions aimed to support people with dementia to adapt and manage their conditions while preserving a sense of self, identity, and social participation. Quinn et al. (2022) report the key areas identified by people with dementia regarding the concept of living well. The key concepts reported are mostly related to psychosocial aspects such as being engaged, having an active lifestyle, preserving positive relationships with others, having a good living situation and environment, having security, getting on with life, being able to get out and about, a positive outlook on life, being able to cope, having independence, and having a purpose in life. As discussed by the authors, all these domains are related to both psychological and social aspects. In the work of Kim and Shin (2023), similar results are reported and four domains of the concept of living well have been identified: physical (maintaining independence and symptoms management); psychological (psychological health, emotional balance, and preservation of a sense of self and identity); social relationships (social relation, community connectivity, support policies).

What emerges from all these conceptualizations is the important role of carers, environment, and context in supporting and promoting the chance of living well with dementia. Despite the consequences of the disease that can undermine the person's abilities, the social environment can play an important role in recognising the strengths and resources of people with dementia, in facilitating their need for independence, and in using the appropriate approach and services to manage symptoms. Similarly, at a psychological level, the empowerment of people with dementia is needed. Being recognised by others, receiving support to cope with challenges, and having trained professionals and available interventions to develop a positive approach are necessary to allow people living with dementia to maintain their quality of life.

Furthermore, the social environment can have an important role in ensuring engagement and participation in community life, preserving social relationships, and supporting inclusion in the social environment. Finally, the health care and welfare systems need to build skills and approaches which are not focused on meeting basic needs exclusively, but also on promoting a more person-centred approach to meet other individual needs such as inclusion, utility, belonging, participation as well as on preserving dignity.

7.4 Social Health and Dementia

In the recent two decades, a significant change occurred in the global approach to dementia. The World Health Organization stated that dementia is a public health priority and a global plan was proposed to tackle the burden of the disease. In many countries, a national plan for dementia has been developed where psychosocial interventions are highly recommended (Chirico et al., 2021). The interventions are not only addressed to manage symptoms but also to promote living well with dementia. Beyond specific interventions directed to people with dementia and their caregivers, a large body of initiatives addressed the issue of stigma and social inclusion. Recently, the promotion of dementia-friendly communities in different countries has aimed to reduce stigma while promoting the social health of people with dementia. The main pillars of the concept of dementia-friendly communities are raising public awareness about dementia, training the public to deal with people with dementia and to facilitate their participation and inclusion, and adapting the social context and environment to the needs and challenges posed by the disease. The dementia-friendly approach aims to involve people with dementia in decisions regarding themselves. This perspective involves not only people with dementia, family caregivers and health care professionals but also public and private sectors such as banks, public services, groceries, and many other sectors.

Social inclusion and participation can be also promoted using specific interventions such as social activities, adapted work opportunities, visiting museums, and so on.

Promoting social health and social inclusion can have different impacts on the journey of people with dementia. It can play a role in the prevention of cognitive decline and in enhancing cognitive reserve (Vernooij-Dassen et al., 2022), but it can also impact the quality of life, well-being, and the excess of dementia-related disability.

7.5   Changing Narratives

Good living with dementia is a complex issue and encompasses different domains of life. The shift in the approach to chronic disease in general, and to dementia in particular, enhances the capability to focus on the experience of the person and of their carers rather than looking only at the disease. To achieve the objective a broad approach is required and different domains need to be addressed.

Certainly, research for a cure is needed, but while waiting for a cure, it is still crucial to support people with dementia and their caregivers. This support can be provided through different actions at individual, family, societal, and governmental levels. To support people with dementia, the recognition of their being a person with values, capacities, and strengths is needed. To achieve this objective, a different narrative of the dementia experience is necessary. Changing narratives, from a negative and helpless one to a more positive and empowering one, can be achieved if the dynamic between individual and society is addressed.

The example of stigma is very meaningful. Public stigma and self-stigma can be seen as an interactive process. What others think, feel, and act toward a specific group is internalised by at least part of the target group. In the case of dementia, negative views have an impact on the experience of the person affected, influencing their quality of life, and their ability to participate in social life, preserve independence, and manage their life. From this perspective, the social health framework including both individual and social-environmental domains can be used as an umbrella concept to advance both research and practice in dementia care.

Acknowledgements Rabih Chattat is grateful for the support of project EPIC (Epistemic Injustice in Healthcare, 2023–2029), generously funded by a Wellcome Discovery Award and led by Havi Carel at the University of Bristol.

REFERENCES

Bodner, E. (2009). On the origins of ageism among older and younger adults. *International Psychogeriatrics, 21*(6), 1003–1014. https://doi.org/10.1017/S104161020999055X. Epub 2009 Jul 21 PMID: 19619389.

Brooker, D. (2007). *Person-Centred dementia care. Making services better Dawn Brooker Person-Centred Dementia Care.* Jessica Kingsley.

Burley, C. V., Casey, A.N., Chenoweth, L., & Brodaty, H. (2021). Reconceptualising behavioral and psychological symptoms of dementia: Views of People Living With Dementia and Families/Care Partners. *Front Psychiatry.* 2021 Aug 16;12:710703.https://doi.org/10.3389/fpsyt.2021.710703. PMID: 34484001; PMCID: PMC8415310.

Butler, R. N. (1969). Age-ism: Another form of bigotry. *The Gerontologist, 9*(4), 243–246.

Chirico, I., Chattat, R., Dostálová, V., Povolná, P., Holmerová, I., de Vugt, M. E., Janssen, N., Dassen, F., Sánchez-Gómez, M. C., García-Peñalvo, F. J., Franco-Martín, M. A., & Ottoboni, G. (2021). The integration of psychosocial care into national dementia strategies across Europe: Evidence from the skills in DEmentia care (SiDECar) project. *International Journal of Environmental Research and Public Health, 18*(7), 3422. https://doi.org/10.3390/ijerph18073422. PMID: 33806158; PMCID: PMC8036745.

Dupuis, S., Wiersma, E., & Loiselle, L. (2012). Pathologizing behavior: Meanings of behaviors in dementia care. *Journal of Aging Studies, 26*, 162–173. https://doi.org/10.1016/j.jaging.2011.12.001

Evans, S. C. (2018). Ageism and dementia. In L. Ayalon & C. Tesch-Römer (Eds.), *Contemporary perspectives on ageism: Vol. 19. International perspectives on aging* (pp. 263–275). Berlin Press.

Huber, M., Knottnerus, J. A., Green, L., van der Horst, H., Jadad, A. R., Kromhout, D., Leonard, B., Lorig, K., Loureiro, M. I., van der Meer, J. W., Schnabel, P., Smith, R., van Weel, C., & Smid, H. (2011, July). How should we define health? *BMJ, 26*(343), d4163. https://doi.org/10.1136/bmj.d4163. PMID: 21791490.

Italian guidelines Diagnosis and treatment of MCI and Dementia. https://www.iss.it/-/snlg-diagnosi-e-trattamento-delle-demenze

Kang, H., & Kim, H. (2022, April 11). Ageism and psychological well-being among older adults: A systematic review. *Gerontology and Geriatric Medicine, 8*, 23337214221087023. https://doi.org/10.1177/23337214221087023. PMID: 35434202; PMCID: PMC9008869.

Kate, S. (2015). Swaffer K. Dementia and prescribed Disengagement[TM]. *Dementia, 14*(1), 3–6. https://doi.org/10.1177/1471301214548136

Kim, J., & Shin, N. (2023). Development of the "living well" concept for older people with dementia. *BMC Geriatrics, 23*, 611. https://doi.org/10.1186/s12877-023-04304-3

Kitwood T. (1987) *Dementia and its pathology: in brain*, mind orsociety? Free Associations *8*, 81–93.

Kitwood T. (1989) *Brain, mind and dementia: with particular ref-erence to Alzheimer's disease*. Ageing and Society *9*, 1–15.

Kitwood T. (1990a) Concern for 'Others'. A New Psychology ofConscience and Morality. Routledge, London, UK.

Kitwood T. (1990b) *The dialetics of dementia: with particular ref-erence to Alzheimer's disease*. Aging and Society 10, 177–196

Kitwood T. (1992) *Quality assurance in dementia care*. GeriatricMedicine, 22, 34–38.

Kitwood T. (1993a) Person and process in dementia. *International Journal of Psychiatry 8*, 541–545.

Kitwood T. (1993b) *Towards a theory of dementia care: the inter-personal process*. Ageing and Society *13*, 51–67.

Kitwood T. (1995) Positive long-term changes in dementia: somepreliminary observations. *Journal of Mental Health 4*, 133–144.

Kitwood T. & Bredin K. (1991) Person to Person: A Guide to the Care of Those With Failing Mental Powers, 2nd edn. Gale CentrePublications, Loughton, UK.

Kitwood T. & Bredin K. (1992) *Towards a theory of dementia care:personhood and well being*. Aging and Society 12, 269–287.

Kitwood, T. (1997). *Dementia reconsidered: The person comes first*. Open University Press, Buckingham, UK

Low, L. F., McGrath, M., Swaffer, K., & Brodaty, H. (2019). Communicating a diagnosis of dementia: A systematic mixed studies review of attitudes and practices of health practitioners. *Dementia, 18*, 2856–2905.

Mariani, E., Vernooij-Dassen, M., Koopmans, R., Engels, Y., & Chattat, R. (2017). Shared decision-making in dementia care planning: Barriers and facilitators in two European countries. (2017). *Aging & Mental Health, 21*(1), 31–39. https://doi.org/10.1080/13607863.2016.1255715. Epub 2016 Nov 21. PMID: 27869501.

NICE guidelines. (2006). https://www.nice.org.uk/guidance/cg42

NICE guidelines. (2018). https://www.nice.org.uk/guidance/ng97

Quinn, C., Pickett, J. A., Litherland, R., Morris, R. G., Martyr, A., Clare L., & On behalf of the IDEAL Programme Team. (2022). Living well with dementia: What is possible and how to promote it. *International Journal of Geriatric Psychiatry, 37*(1). https://doi.org/10.1002/gps.5627. https://doi.org/10.1002/gps.5627. Epub 2021 Oct 13. PMID: 34564897; PMCID: PMC9292841.

Sabat, S. R., & Lee, J. M. (2012). Relatedness among people diagnosed with dementia: Social cognition and the possibility of friendship. *Dementia, 11*(3), 315–327. https://doi.org/10.1177/1471301211421069

Samtani, S., Mahalingam, G., Lam, B., Lipnicki, D., Lima-Costa, M., Blay, S., et al. (2022). Associations between social connections and cognition: A global collaborative individual participant data meta-analysis. *The Lancet Healthy Longevity, 3*, e740–e753. https://doi.org/10.1016/S2666-7568(22)00199-443

Seifert, I., Wiegelmann, H., Lenart-Bugla, M., Łuc, M., Pawłowski, M., Rouwette, E., et al. (2022). Mapping the complexity of dementia: Factors influencing cognitive function at the onset of dementia. *BMC Geriatrics 22*, 507. https://doi.org/10.1186/s12877-022-02955-2

Stokes, G. (2000). Challenging Behaviour in Dementia: A Person-Centred Approach (1st ed.). Routledge. https://doi.org/10.4324/9781315168715

Van den Bossche, P., & Schoenmakers, B. (2022). The impact of dementia's sffiliate stigma on the mental health of relatives: A cross section survey. *Frontiers in Psychology, 20*(12), 789105. https://doi.org/10.3389/fpsyg.2021.789105.PMID:35126240;PMCID:PMC8811187

Vernooij-Dassen, M., Moniz-Cook, E., Verhey, F., Chattat, R., Woods, B., Meiland, F., Franco, M., Holmerova, I., Orrell, M., & de Vugt, M. (2021). Bridging the divide between biomedical and psychosocial approaches in dementia research: The 2019 INTERDEM manifesto. *Aging & Mental Health, 25*(2), 206–212. https://doi.org/10.1080/13607863.2019.1693968. Epub 2019 Nov 26 PMID: 31771338.

Vernooij-Dassen M, Verspoor E, Samtani S, Sachdev PS, Ikram MA, Vernooij MW, Hubers C, Chattat R, Lenart-Bugla M, Rymaszewska J, Szczesniak D, Brodaty H, Welmer AK, Maddock J, van der Velpen IF, Wiegelmann H, Marseglia A, Richards M, Melis R, de Vugt M, Moniz-Cook E, Jeon

YH, Perry M, Wolf-Ostermann K. Recognition of social health: A conceptual framework in the context of dementia research. Front Psychiatry. (2022) Dec 15;13:1052009. https://doi.org/10.3389/fpsyt.2022.1052009. PMID: 36590639; PMCID: PMC9798783.

Wollney, E. N., Armstrong, M. J., Bedenfield, N., Rosselli, M., Curiel-Cid, R. E., Kitaigorodsky, M., Levy, X., & Bylund, C. L. (2022). Barriers and best practices in disclosing a dementia diagnosis: A clinician interview study. *Health Services Insights*, 5(15), 11786329221141828. https://doi.org/10.1177/11786329221141829.PMID:36506598;PMCID:PMC9729996

Woods, B., Arosio, F., Diaz, A., Gove, D., Holmerová, I., Kinnaird, L., Mátlová, M., Okkonen, E., Possenti, M., Roberts, J., Salmi, A., van den Buuse, S., Werkman, W., & Georges, J. (2019). Timely diagnosis of dementia? Family carers' experiences in 5 European countries. *International Psychogeriatrics*, 34(1), 114–121. https://doi.org/10.1002/gps.4997. Epub 2018 Oct 9. PMID: 30246266; PMCID: PMC6586062.

Yates, J., Stanyon, M., Samra, R., & Clare, L. (2021). Challenges in disclosing and receiving a diagnosis of dementia: A systematic review of practice from the perspectives of people with dementia, carers, and healthcare professionals. *International Psychogeriatrics*, 33(11), 1161–1192. https://doi.org/10.1017/S1041610221000119. Epub 2021 Mar 17 PMID: 33726880.

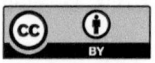

CHAPTER 8

Ameliorating Epistemic Injustice with Digital Health Technologies

Elisabetta Lalumera ⓘ

Abstract This chapter discusses the potential of digital phenotyping to ameliorate epistemic injustice in mental health. Digital phenotyping, which analyses behavioural patterns from user data or smart devices, shows promise in improving mental health care. Whilst concerns exist that it may exacerbate epistemic injustice by overshadowing individual experiences, the chapter presents a different viewpoint. Through a fictional case study, digital phenotyping is portrayed as aiding individuals seeking help by offering more accurate evidence and supporting shared decision-making. The objection that digital technology overrides personal claims is countered by arguing against absolute epistemic priority for any diagnostic tool in medicine. The chapter acknowledges the need for technological advancements and ethical considerations but maintains a positive outlook on the future of digital phenotyping in mental healthcare.

E. Lalumera (✉)
Department for Life Quality Studies, University of Bologna, Rimini, Italy
e-mail: elisabetta.lalumera@unibo.it

© The Author(s) 2025   141
L. Bortolotti (ed.), *Epistemic Justice in Mental Healthcare*,
https://doi.org/10.1007/978-3-031-68881-2_8

Keywords Epistemic injustice · Digital phenotyping · Mental health · ADHD · Diagnosis · Medical technology · Predictive models · Clinical decision-making

8.1   Digital Phenotyping and Epistemic Justice

Digital phenotyping involves the identification of behavioural patterns (phenotypes) from digital data entered by users or recorded by their smart devices, such as watches. In mental healthcare, digital phenotyping holds promise for supporting diagnosis, monitoring recovery, and customizing therapeutic approaches (Insel, 2018; Torous et al., 2016). Whilst its widespread clinical implementation remains nascent, numerous technologies and applications are already available for various conditions, including depression, psychosis, child and adult ADHD, complemented by recommendations and guidelines from scientific societies (Bufano et al., 2023; Kalman et al., 2023).

Given this context, it is not premature to address a philosophical question about digital phenotyping in psychiatry: is it conceptually compatible with epistemic justice, which entails giving individuals seeking care due credibility? Currently, the predominant trend in literature is to consider digital phenotyping unfavourably, implying that technology may worsen epistemic injustice by potentially overshadowing or undercutting individual voices and experiences in favour of clinical judgement and algorithmic decisions (Birk et al., 2021; Slack & Barclay, 2023). However, in this chapter, I argue that digital phenotyping may actually alleviate epistemic injustice in psychiatry. I suggest that it possesses this potential in various ways, including reducing systemic interpretive injustice, addressing biases underpinning testimonial epistemic injustice amongst healthcare professionals, and empowering users to seek help and correct ineffective or harmful treatment paths.

It's essential to clarify that my argument does not assert the inherent goodness of all digital phenotyping technologies in psychiatry. Digital phenotyping inherits all of the challenges associated with digital technologies—including ethical data privacy legislation, attention to potential biases in algorithms, and systematic social action to prevent them from contributing to the increasing of health inequities caused by the technological gap (Birk et al., 2021; Quinn et al., 2022)—therefore, many prerequisites must be met, before they can be considered ethically viable. My aim is rather to establish the conceptual compatibility between digital phenotyping and epistemic justice in psychiatry, provided that such prerequisites are met. Achieving this compatibility necessitates the conscious calibration of digital phenotyping solutions in collaboration with persons undergoing treatment and specialists, acknowledging their limitations, potentials, and specific epistemic roles within the diagnostic and treatment process.

The structure of my chapter is as follows: I begin by providing a brief overview of the potential benefits of digital phenotyping in psychiatry, building on previously published reviews. Following that, I give an illustrated scenario—a vignette—to demonstrate how digital phenotyping could reduce epistemic injustice in a context of mental healthcare. In the third section, I address one of the arguments for the conclusion that digital phenotyping exacerbates epistemic injustice in psychiatry. Worries have been expressed about how people might not recognize themselves in algorithmic diagnoses or descriptions of their psychological states, and about the potential negative effects of risk assessments produced by this kind of technology (Pozzi, 2023; Slack & Barclay, 2023). To these issues, I respond that when an individual's claim conflicts with the predictive or diagnostic verdict of digital technology, epistemic injustice occurs only when the tool's output is given absolute epistemic priority. Instead, I argue that epistemic priority in medicine must always be relative and proportional to the accuracy of the instruments, and hence, the criticism is based on an unsound principle. Moreover, no technological device should be given absolute priority in decision-making, independently of its accuracy.

8.2   DIGITAL PHENOTYPING IN MENTAL HEALTH

In this section, I will briefly describe digital phenotyping and its current prospects and applications in mental health. Let's start by clarifying a few terms. A behavioural phenotype is a collection of observable behaviours displayed by a person or group in reaction to internal or external stimuli. These behaviours might include a variety of acts, reactions, and patterns, such as cognitive processes, emotional responses, social interactions, and movements. Numerous factors, such as development, environment, heredity, and individual differences, affect behavioural phenotypes. In the context of mental health, behavioural phenotypes are key for understanding, diagnosing, and treating conditions because they provide insights into an individual's psychological functioning and well-being. This is because the treatment of mental health is currently based on watching and analysing behaviour, as there are no biological or genetic biomarkers for psychiatric nosological conditions like those for oncological or metabolic diseases, and some believe there will never be (Wolfers et al., 2018). A behavioural phenotype is "digital" when it is created from the data obtained from a person's interaction with their smartphone or smartwatch, computer, or other wearable technology (Onnela & Rauch, 2016; Torous et al., 2016). The "data" in digital phenotyping are categorized into active and passive. Active data necessitate user engagement, such as completing questionnaires about mood on one's own smartwatch. Passive data are collected from sensors and logs without any burden on the subject. They encompass metrics like the number of text messages sent, accelerometry, and geolocation. Biometric data such as heart rate, sleep patterns, and skin conductance made available with smartwatches and other wearables also belong to this group (Onnela, 2021).

This is essentially how a digital phenotyping technology operates. After data are uploaded to a server or device, they undergoe preprocessing, including cleaning, to prepare them for further analysis. Machine learning algorithms are then employed to identify predictive behavioural features and other biomarkers from these raw data sets. The main challenge lies in developing an algorithm capable of making valid connections between features such as the frequency of sent messages or heightened heart rate, and an individual's psychological state, such as anxiety. Ultimately, the goal representation of the person's mental state and functioning is created by integrating the identified features with electronic self-reports and other active data. The final crucial stage for digital phenotyping in psychiatry stage is clinical implementation, that is, adoption of a valid procedure that connects detection of changes in the digital phenotype with various interventions. This process, known as "closing the loop," involves actions such as preventing relapse, identifying non-response to treatment, delivering timely intervention, suggesting a diagnosis, revising an existing diagnosis, or uncovering comorbidities (Williamson, 2023).

Let's briefly see why digital phenotyping should bring benefits to the treatment of mental health conditions. According to its advocates, digital phenotyping has important epistemic advantages over other types of behavioural observations and evaluations. First, digital phenotyping is an ecological observation, which means it captures the individual in their daily existence (Huckvale et al., 2019). Traditionally, the evaluation interview for a psychiatric or psychological visit is brief, structured, and may not always reflect the person's typical condition in daily life (for example, they may be calmer or more upset since they are attending a medical consultation). More specifically, in psychiatry, retrospective questionnaires conducted by clinicians and self-reports are considered the gold standard. Unfortunately, retrospective measures are susceptible to memory distortions and may show how people reconstruct the past rather than how they experienced it, and current mood is likely to alter the information recalled (Onnela & Rauch, 2016). Moreover, retrospective recollection of average levels of mood or symptoms may be more challenging than considering the present time, especially for people with distressing conditions. Digital phenotyping could address this problem. It can also "expand the psychiatrist's sensory" by including information not generally available in an interview, like as a person's heart rate or the number of texts they've sent (Williamson, 2023).

Given that mental health issues are deeply influenced by context and social factors, it's crucial to gather data in a way that reflects these ecological dynamics. Ecological Momentary Assessment (EMA) is a well-established method for assessing behaviour and emotions in real time ("in situ"), widely used across medicine, psychiatry, and psychology (Stone & Shiffman, 1994). However, traditional EMA requires individuals to actively respond to questions about their state at various times throughout the day, demanding their involvement, effort, and cognitive processing. The shift to digital introduces passive data entry, which, unlike active EMA, occurs continuously and effortlessly, without placing any burden on the individual. This transition to passive data entry marks a significant advancement in data collection methods, offering a more ecologically valid and less intrusive approach to understanding mental health dynamics (Onnela, 2021).

Attention-deficit/hyperactivity disorder (ADHD) makes a good example of how to exploit this feature of digital phenotyping. ADHD is defined by dynamic symptoms, including hyperactivity, inattention, and impulsivity, as well as emotion dysregulation. Although much research has been conducted to investigate between-subject differences (how patients with ADHD differ from healthy controls or patients with other disorders), little is known about the relationship between symptoms and triggers, which could help us better understand their causes and consequences. A study financed by the European Union analysed e-diaries apps in the monitoring of ADHD, with the aim of understanding the temporal relationships between symptoms and environmental triggers in an ecologically accurate manner (Koch et al., 2021).

A further epistemic benefit of digital phenotyping is personalization. Data are collected and analysed at the individual rather than group level. Group-level data are useful for determining, for example, how the prevalence of a pattern of behaviour or illness varies with sociodemographic factors, but they cannot be used to make inferences about individuals without committing ecological fallacy, which is making inferences about individuals based on inferences about the group to which those individuals belong. "Individual-level" in digital phenotyping also means that many data analyses focus on within-person changes over time (Bickman et al., 2016). At the conceptual level, this resurrects the idea of Georges Canguilhem, who argued that every person is their own norm and that the concept of normal and abnormal is strictly unique (Canguilhem, 2012). We find here a theme that defies the biomedical paradigm, based on epidemiological or clinical evidence supplied by trials at group level.

In spite of the abundance of new studies, it is crucial to realize that, at the time of writing, digital phenotyping in psychiatry is more of a promise than a reliable instrument (Anmella et al., 2022; Engelmann & Wackers, 2022). There are technical challenges—real-world data obtained from smartwatches, smartphones, wearables, and human–computer interactions are often noisy, patchy, and substantial in size, and unlike in fields like medical imaging or genomics, there is no standardized method for analysing data from digital devices (Williamson, 2023). Moreover, systematizing and validating digital phenotyping tools necessitates collaborative, reproducible, and transparent studies, whereas we still find ourselves in a situation where digital phenotyping is tested in specific applications, via small studies, and works with algorithms and devices that are very different, making them incomparable (Bufano et al., 2023). Finally, there is currently no consensus on how to close the loop in psychiatric digital phenotyping, that is, how to respond to the evidence provided by the tool—a point I will also elaborate on in the fourth section below (Huckvale et al., 2019). In sum, effectively harnessing the potential of digital phenotyping in mental healthcare requires a blend of technical, legal, clinical, and methodological expertise to translate promise into tangible benefits (Kalman et al., 2023).

8.3   Ameliorating Epistemic
Injustice with Digital Phenotyping

I have just illustrated that there is still much work to be done before digital phenotyping becomes routine in mental healthcare. However, most of the methodological and conceptual aspects of these new tools are sufficiently evident to allow for a priori assessment of some structural traits. For example, as seen above, it has been claimed that they may structurally provide certain epistemic advantages when compared to traditional assessment tools in mental healthcare. But where does digital phenotyping stand in terms of epistemic risks, and specifically, the risk of epistemic injustice, or not giving the correct credence to the person's point of view in the care interaction, because of prejudices about the group to which they belong? The research in the humanities appears to agree on the negative verdict: digital phenotyping is or will be another tool of epistemic injustice in psychiatry (Engelmann & Wackers, 2022). Here, however, I'd want to argue the opposite of that. In this section, I present a fictitious example, a vignette, to show how digital phenotyping could mitigate epistemic injustice. The meaning of the example is as follows: digital phenotyping could be a tool to be believed and validated in the request for help, care, and even a more specific diagnosis. For the construction of my vignette, I rely on recent research on so-called high-functioning adult ADHD, a somewhat under researched and underdiagnosed condition (Crook & McDowall, 2023; Hoben & Hesson, 2021).

Meet A, a woman in her forties, juggling the roles of a university professor, a mother to two children from different relationships, and a partner to someone living in another city. Despite her outward appearance of good health and well-being, A's life is fraught with financial struggles, including significant expenses from divorces and accidents for which she was at fault. She often receives fines for driving infractions and once overlooked declaring income from a translation job. Despite her modest lifestyle, she occasionally splurges on unnecessary purchases, sometimes even going beyond her means to indulge in holidays she can't afford for herself and her children. In her professional life, A has battled feelings of inadequacy and unreliability, often feeling as though her ideas slip through her fingers and struggling to meet deadlines. She's been in therapy for years due to episodes of depression and a previous diagnosis of borderline personality disorder, which later specialists refuted. Over the years, A continues to grapple with dissatisfaction and seeks answers to her challenges.

One day, whilst reading, A stumbles upon a description of ADHD symptoms in adult women. Intriguingly, many of the traits outlined resonate with her own experiences. Eager to gain clarity, she schedules a psychiatric evaluation to confirm her suspicions. However, the outcome is not what A anticipates. The doctor explains that whilst A's own story suggests the possibility of ADHD, her performance in assessment tests for her executive functions is average. Moreover, A's functionality in her career and personal life, including her role as a professor and her responsibilities as a parent and partner, seems incongruent with such a diagnosis. Overall, according to the doctor, the typical phenotype of adult ADHD starkly contrast with A's outward appearance of health and stability and with her overall success. This puts an end to the possibility of confirming an ADHD diagnosis, and A goes back home with an illness with no name.

I would like to add that A's doctor should not be considered particularly arrogant or uninformed here. It is very difficult to diagnose ADHD in adult individuals, especially if they have a high IQ or cognitive abilities that systematically compensate for their difficulties in executive functions (Milioni et al., 2017).

Years go by, and advancements in technology lead to the validation of a digital phenotype for adult ADHD. A, upon learning about this breakthrough, collaborates with her therapist to explore this possibility. She downloads the necessary app and undergoes testing, revealing patterns of impulsive spending, bouts of intense or "hyper" focus, and prolonged periods of unproductivity—details that eluded detection in her initial assessment. The digital phenotype, in conjunction with traditional diagnostic tests and A's own insights, undergoes careful analysis by her therapist. Ultimately, A receives a diagnosis that aligns with her self-identification, providing her with the validation she has long sought regarding her life experiences.

Let us see how, in this fictional case, digital phenotyping helped A. Because A was observed in greater detail by the technology, an appropriate diagnosis was possible. The psychiatrist now has access to a variety of new and diverse information, whereas previously the psychiatrist's assessment of A was limited to the conversation and the patient's appearance and behaviour during visits. This material exposes A's struggles in life and at work, which were previously concealed by the fact that A was consistently able to make up for them with respectable levels of success in both her career and relationships. A now has proof of her particular pattern of suffering, which the therapist can validate, thanks to digital phenotyping. A gains insight into their experience and life narrative and can initiate targeted treatment, including medication-assisted therapy or psychotherapy grounded in fresh information. Essentially, in this case, digital phenotyping has done more good than harm, as in any case where a more accurate diagnostic tool or support is introduced in medicine—for example, imaging technologies that accurately locate and monitor tumour progression and response to therapy—with the additional benefit, in this specific case, of validating the illness claims that previously were dismissed. In addition, the therapist can easily understand and trust this way of validating illness claims.

Now we must address the key point, which is that this greater good than harm is specifically aimed at alleviating epistemic injustice. We know from A's fictional case that her former therapist did not accept her suggestion to rename her illness as ADHD—a term that had never been suggested to A in her career as a healthcare user. In this, A's credibility was harmed and diminished. To be a victim of epistemic injustice, one must, nevertheless, be more than just someone who is not taken seriously or who is not given credit for their epistemic contributions; not all mistakes in credibility assessment qualify as epistemic injustices (Fricker, 2007). We're interested in the phenomena in which someone is not believed, listened to, or understood because of a bias or stereotype about the type of person they are.

Does A fit this description? It does, in at least two ways—as we can see if we examine attentively, there is overlapping injustice regarding A's knowledge capability. The first and most evident stereotype she falls prey to is the more familiar from the epistemic injustice in healthcare literature: A is undervalued in her capacity to aid in the diagnosis by providing information that differs from what the therapist gathers from questionnaires and assessments because she is a sick person, and she is viewed a non-expert by the therapist. Crichton, Kidd, and Carel provide a thorough illustration of this particular form of epistemic injustice committed by mental health professionals against people seeking care, and the idea is carried through in a number of other publications (Crichton et al., 2017; Drożdżowicz, 2021; Houlders et al., 2021; Spencer, 2023).

I would add that A is a victim of epistemic injustice because of an additional stereotype that undermines her credibility more subtly and elusively. It is the misconception that people who are prima facie good-looking, with an adequate income, and with decent relationship and emotional achievement cannot be unwell, i.e. cannot bring genuine experiences of struggle and suffering. Insofar as the therapist's two intersecting stereotypes undermine A's authority, we can acknowledge that A is a victim of epistemic injustice. However, to the degree that the app's digital phenotyping has made a successful diagnosis possible, this technology has also helped to ameliorate the testimonial epistemic injustice committed against A.

I'd like to briefly expand on the point about the "positive" stereotype that the app contributes to mitigating. Since adult ADHD is now receiving more attention, studies have shown that one of the barriers to receiving a proper diagnosis is precisely the perception of sanity from the therapist's part, which can occur when adults with ADHD have compensatory mechanisms that enable them to function—if not thrive—despite their condition (Crook & McDowall, 2023; Hoben & Hesson, 2021). But stereotyping is not the only bias that psychiatrists and therapists, like other healthcare practitioners, are susceptible to during the diagnostic process (Blumenthal-Barby & Krieger, 2015). Another cognitive bias that is relevant here is anchoring, in which the therapist bases a diagnosis on the first impression of a person. In A's case, the first therapist that dismissed A's suggestion of an ADHD diagnosis could be described as anchoring to A's prima facie appearance (A appeared healthy) and therefore disregarding the specific pattern of pain that she was attempting to express. Anchoring in this case reinforces stereotyping and produces epistemic injustice. One of the possible advantages of technology-aided diagnosis is precisely to mitigate cognitive biases such as stereotyping and anchoring, in psychiatry as elsewhere (Mouchabac et al., 2021). In as much as these are crucial to testimonial epistemic injustice, digital phenotyping can contribute to ameliorate it.

It is also necessary to consider interpretative epistemic injustice in order to determine whether and how digital phenotyping can have an ameliorating role. Interpretive or hermeneutical epistemic injustice arises when a structurally dominating group fails to acquire the conceptual tools to make sense of the experiences of people from less dominant epistemic groups and to include them equally in the interchange of knowledge—in healthcare, when therapists do not engage in finding out the resources to understand some group of people's illness claims (Carel & Kidd, 2017; Medina, 2017). If and when digital phenotyping works, as illustrated in the invented example of A, it provides a detailed and complete behavioural trace of psychological states that, on the one hand, is as close to the complexity of personal experience as possible, whilst also using a language that the therapist understands and has already been translated, so to speak, into an intersubjective code. In this way, digital phenotyping fills a gap in the therapist's understanding and, as a result, mitigates interpretative epistemic injustice.

8.4 Epistemic Injustice and Absolute Epistemic Priority

As previously said, there is agreement in sociology and philosophy of medicine that AI-based technologies and digital phenotyping are tools that exacerbate epistemic unfair treatment towards patients rather than alleviate it. In this chapter, I will discuss one of the objections that has been made, which offers an example that is exactly comparable to my own with rA and the ADHD app. The critique is that the patient may not recognize themselves in the phenotype, symptom description, diagnostic verdict, disease risk assessment, or overall output provided by the algorithm. When this occurs, technology becomes a tool of epistemic oppression in the hands of doctors. Melissa McCradden and colleagues (McCradden et al., 2023) provide this example. A person visits the psychiatric emergency department with distressing suicide thoughts, low mood, and anxiety. A predictive AI model built to assess acute risk deprioritizes urgent care because there is a low possibility of imminent demand. The model's decisions are influenced by a borderline personality disorder diagnosis. The patient's assertions of increased danger are therefore minimized, resulting in a referral to outpatient care.

According to McCradden and colleagues, this is an example of epistemic injustice, where the person's clear call for assistance is ignored owing to algorithmic prediction, as the model's verdict takes precedence over the patient's urgent care plea. The same claim is made by Giorgia Pozzi, elaborating on a fictional example of a person in need who is denied opioid prescription because she is incorrectly categorized as high-risk of addiction by a predictive model (Pozzi, 2023).

This kind of fictional examples is diametrically opposed to the one I described above, in the sense that for A, the output of digital technology (in this case, the digital phenotype) is supporting evidence, whereas here it is proof against the patient's claim. Likewise, whilst technology could ameliorate epistemic unfairness in example A, it actually enhances it here.

One may be tempted to draw a simple conclusion: perhaps digital technology and digital phenotyping are tools for mitigating epistemic injustice when they support the first-person narrative of the individual seeking help and means for epistemic injustice when they undermine it. If we follow this reasoning, we must conclude that digital technology in mental health is neutral in terms of epistemic injustice, as it sometimes mitigates and sometimes exacerbates it.

However, this conclusion would not address our original conceptual question: Does digital phenotyping support or undermine epistemic justice, before we examine how frequently the technology's findings correspond with an individual's own testimony?

Let us try another way. As pointed out in both papers under consideration, an epistemic injustice arises in the application of digital technology because the clinician considers this much more than any other source of evidence, particularly the claims of the person seeking assistance. In other words, the diagnostic tool's evidence is given absolute epistemic priority. This attribution of absolute epistemic priority to the machine's verdict is described as a very likely risk (a possibility) (McCradden et al., 2023) but also as something that is already happening (a fact) (Pozzi, 2023).

Given the lack of data on the usage of predictive digital technologies, it is critical to return to the conceptual level in this discussion. Certainly, it is possible that absolute epistemic priority is given to a diagnostic or predictive tool in medicine, but from a conceptual and normative perspective, this is not justified either epistemically or ethically. Let us see why, in clinical assessment and diagnosis, such an absolute epistemic priority principle is, at the very least, contentious. To begin with, all medical technologies, whether predictive or diagnostic, have an accuracy level that essentially represents their capacity for error-free performance (Deeks et al., 2023). The accuracy of diagnostic tests and technologies varies greatly, especially without the use of artificial intelligence or the complex field of psychiatry. A clinical test performed by an orthopaedic surgeon or physiotherapist to determine whether there is a meniscus damage (knee joint) typically has an accuracy of about 70%, whereas a lab pregnancy test has an accuracy of 99% (Shekarchi et al., 2020). If we take accuracy into consideration, it makes sense to give the results of a pregnancy test epistemic priority above the statements of someone claiming, say, that they are not pregnant. It makes considerably less sense and is not justifiable to give priority to a clinical test in the case of a meniscus injury over the patient's medical history or the information they supply. Essentially, my point here is that any test or diagnostic technology has a relative epistemic priority and this should be based on how accurate it is—a point acknowledged by (Carel & Kidd, 2014).

There is another crucial step to make: although a test or extremely accurate diagnostic technology may legitimately have epistemic priority over a patient's claim in a clinical assessment or even diagnosis, it is not the same thing to state that the diagnostic tool can dictate the clinical decision. The last five decades of bioethics have taught us, at the very least, that the individual receiving medical care and the healthcare provider must always collaborate to make the clinical decision. If a highly accurate imaging test reveals to the orthopaedic surgeon and person B that there is a substantial lesion, and we agree that this test is the best approach to determine what is going on with B's meniscus, it will still be B, together with the healthcare professional, who decides what to do, whether surgery, other types of interventions, or simply going home hopping on the other foot.

Let us return to digital phenotyping and other AI-based diagnostic and prediction solutions for mental health. For the time being, none are as accurate as a pregnancy test, and there are strong indications that none will ever be. As a result, it is unlikely that we will be able to justify giving the results of these diagnostic tools epistemic priority. Moreover, it is impossible to defend giving the digital phenotype or the risk predictor's output absolute priority in clinical decision-making, as is the case with all clinical and predictive testing in medicine. Technologies can be useful decision-making tools, and the therapist will consider them based on their accuracy and validity. However, ultimately, the choice on what to do must come from the interaction between the therapist and the individual in care.

We now have a response for the criticism of McCradden and colleagues and Pozzi. Their concern was that when the algorithm does not validate the claim of the person seeking assistance, it will inevitably override the person's voice. The response is that the algorithm will only trump persons' voices if we grant it absolute epistemic priority and decision-making authority. However, the former should be dependent on the accuracy and validity of the technological tool, and the latter is, to put it simply, always ethically and procedurally inappropriate in clinical encounters. As a result, the psychiatric emergency case presented as example of epistemic injustice is rather a case of bad medicine, in which the shortcomings and functions of the digital technology are not adequately understood.

8.5   LOOKING AT THE FUTURE WITH OPTIMISM

In this chapter, I have provided reasons to respond positively to the question: can a digital technology like digital phenotyping mitigate epistemic injustice in mental health? I have presented a hypothetical case in which the output of the technology becomes an ally for the person seeking help to defend their claim, as it represents them more faithfully, expands the evidence traditionally available to the clinician, and easily integrates into shared decision-making processes. The example demonstrates a conceptual possibility, the realization of which depends factually on the maturation of appropriate technologies in terms of both accuracy and ethical and legislative levels. The hope is that these technologies can mature in the desired direction.

I have considered the objection that digital phenotyping and risk prediction models in mental health are tools of epistemic injustice because they de facto minimize the patient's claim by providing a type of evidence that takes absolute epistemic priority not only in the person's assessment, but also in decision-making. I replied that if the absolute epistemic priority of digital technologies in diagnosis and medical decision-making were justifiable, then digital phenotyping in mental health would be incompatible with epistemic justice and, consequently, could not contribute to it. However, this principle is not defensible in any area of medicine. The fact that clinicians and the system may misapply predictive technologies in mental health is a possibility, but the idea that they must misapply them due to conceptual necessity is a conclusion that does not follow. We must not confuse, in philosophy, the realm of empirical possibilities with the conceptual realm, and bad medicine with bad tools.

Acknowledgements Elisabetta Lalumera acknowledges the support of project EPIC (Epistemic Injustice in Healthcare, 2023–2029), generously funded by a Wellcome Discovery Award and led by Havi Carel at the University of Bristol, and of the Italian Complementary National Plan PNC-I. 1 Research initiatives for innovative technologies and pathways in the health and welfare sector, D.D. 931 of 06/06/2022, DARE—DigitAl lifelong pRevEntion initiative, code PNC0000002, CUP B53C22006450001.

References

Anmella, G., Faurholt-Jepsen, M., Hidalgo-Mazzei, D., Radua, J., Passos, I. C., Kapczinski, F., Minuzzi, L., Alda, M., Meier, S., Hajek, T., Ballester, P., Birmaher, B., Hafeman, D., Goldstein, T., Brietzke, E., Duffy, A., Haarman, B., Lopez-Jaramillo, C., Yatham, L. N., ... Kessing, L. V. (2022). Smartphone-based interventions in bipolar disorder: Systematic review and meta-analyses of efficacy. A position paper from the International Society for Bipolar Disorders (ISBD) Big Data Task Force. *Bipolar Disorders, 24*(6), 580–614. https://doi.org/10.1111/bdi.13243

Bickman, L., Lyon, A. R., & Wolpert, M. (2016). Achieving precision mental health through effective assessment, monitoring, and feedback processes. *Administration and Policy in Mental Health and Mental Health Services Research, 43*(3), 271–276. https://doi.org/10.1007/s10488-016-0718-5

Birk, R., Lavis, A., Lucivero, F., & Samuel, G. (2021). For what it's worth. Unearthing the values embedded in digital phenotyping for mental health. *Big Data & Society, 8*(2), 20539517211047319. https://doi.org/10.1177/20539517211047319

Blumenthal-Barby, J. S., & Krieger, H. (2015). Cognitive biases and heuristics in medical decision making: A critical review using a systematic search strategy. *Medical Decision Making, 35*(4), 539–557. https://doi.org/10.1177/0272989X14547740

Bufano, P., Laurino, M., Said, S., Tognetti, A., & Menicucci, D. (2023). Digital phenotyping for monitoring mental disorders: Systematic review. *Journal of Medical Internet Research, 25*(1), e46778. https://doi.org/10.2196/46778

Canguilhem, G. (2012). *On the normal and the pathological*. Springer Science & Business Media.

Carel, H., & Kidd, I. J. (2014). Epistemic injustice in healthcare: A philosophial analysis. *Medicine, Health Care, and Philosophy, 17*(4), 529–540. https://doi.org/10.1007/s11019-014-9560-2

Carel, H., & Kidd, I. J. (2017). *Epistemic injustice in medicine and healthcare*. Routledge.

Crichton, P., Carel, H., & Kidd, I. J. (2017). Epistemic injustice in psychiatry. *BJPsych Bulletin, 41*(2), 65–70. https://doi.org/10.1192/pb.bp.115.050682

Crook, T., & McDowall, A. (2023). Paradoxical career strengths and successes of ADHD adults: An evolving narrative. *Journal of Work-Applied Management, ahead-of-print* (ahead-of-print). https://doi.org/10.1108/JWAM-05-2023-0048

Deeks, J. J., Bossuyt, P. M., Leeflang, M. M., & Takwoingi, Y. (2023). *Cochrane handbook for systematic reviews of diagnostic test accuracy*. Wiley.

Drożdżowicz, A. (2021). Epistemic injustice in psychiatric practice: Epistemic duties and the phenomenological approach. *Journal of Medical Ethics, 47*(12), e69–e69. https://doi.org/10.1136/medethics-2020-106679

Engelmann, L., & Wackers, G. (2022). Digital phenotyping—Editorial. *Big Data & Society, 9*(2), 20539517221113776. https://doi.org/10.1177/205 39517221113775

Fricker, M. (2007). *Epistemic injustice: Power and the ethics of knowing.* Clarendon Press.

Hoben, J., & Hesson, J. (2021). Invisible lives: Using autoethnography to explore the experiences of academics living with Attention Deficit Hyperactivity Disorder (ADHD). *New Horizons in Adult Education & Human Resource Development, 33*(1), 37–50. https://doi.org/10.1002/nha3.20304

Houlders, J. W., Bortolotti, L., & Broome, M. R. (2021). Threats to epistemic agency in young people with unusual experiences and beliefs. *Synthese, 199*(3), 7689–7704. https://doi.org/10.1007/s11229-021-03133-4

Huckvale, K., Venkatesh, S., & Christensen, H. (2019). Toward clinical digital phenotyping: A timely opportunity to consider purpose, quality, and safety. *NPJ Digital Medicine, 2*(1), 1–11. https://doi.org/10.1038/s41746-019-0166-1

Insel, T. (2018). Digital phenotyping: A global tool for psychiatry. *World Psychiatry: Official Journal of the World Psychiatric Association (WPA), 17*(3), 276–277. https://doi.org/10.1002/wps.20550

Kalman, J. L., Burkhardt, G., Samochowiec, J., Gebhard, C., Dom, G., John, M., Kilic, O., Kurimay, T., Lien, L., Schouler-Ocak, M., Vidal, D. P., Wiser, J., Gaebel, W., Volpe, U., & Falkai, P. (2023). Digitalising mental health care: Practical recommendations from the European Psychiatric Association. *European Psychiatry, 67*(1), e4. https://doi.org/10.1192/j.eurpsy.2023.2466

Koch, E. D., Moukhtarian, T. R., Skirrow, C., Bozhilova, N., Asherson, P., & Ebner-Priemer, U. W. (2021). Using e-diaries to investigate ADHD—State-of-the-art and the promising feature of just-in-time-adaptive interventions. *Neuroscience & Biobehavioral Reviews, 127*, 884–898. https://doi.org/10.1016/j.neubiorev.2021.06.002

McCradden, M., Hui, K., & Buchman, D. Z. (2023). Evidence, ethics and the promise of artificial intelligence in psychiatry. *Journal of Medical Ethics, 49*(8), 573–579. https://doi.org/10.1136/jme-2022-108447

Medina, J. (2017). *Varieties of hermeneutical injustice 1.* Routledge.

Milioni, A. L. V., Chaim, T. M., Cavallet, M., de Oliveira, N. M., Annes, M., dos Santos, B., Louzã, M., da Silva, M. A., Miguel, C. S., Serpa, M. H., Zanetti, M. V., Busatto, G., & Cunha, P. J. (2017). High IQ may "mask" the diagnosis of ADHD by compensating for deficits in executive functions in treatment-Naïve Adults With ADHD. *Journal of Attention Disorders, 21*(6), 455–464. https://doi.org/10.1177/1087054714554933

Mouchabac, S., Conejero, I., Lakhlifi, C., Msellek, I., Malandain, L., Adrien, V., Ferreri, F., Millet, B., Bonnot, O., Bourla, A., & Maatoug, R. (2021).

Improving clinical decision-making in psychiatry: Implementation of digital phenotyping could mitigate the influence of patient's and practitioner's individual cognitive biases. *Dialogues in Clinical Neuroscience, 23*(1), 52–61. https://doi.org/10.1080/19585969.2022.2042165

Onnela, J.-P. (2021). Opportunities and challenges in the collection and analysis of digital phenotyping data. *Neuropsychopharmacology, 46*(1), 45–54. https://doi.org/10.1038/s41386-020-0771-3

Onnela, J.-P., & Rauch, S. L. (2016). Harnessing smartphone-based digital phenotyping to enhance behavioral and mental health. *Neuropsychopharmacology, 41*(7), 1691–1696. https://doi.org/10.1038/npp.2016.7

Pozzi, G. (2023). Automated opioid risk scores: A case for machine learning-induced epistemic injustice in healthcare. *Ethics and Information Technology, 25*(1), 3. https://doi.org/10.1007/s10676-023-09676-z

Quinn, T. P., Jacobs, S., Senadeera, M., Le, V., & Coghlan, S. (2022). The three ghosts of medical AI: Can the black-box present deliver? *Artificial Intelligence in Medicine, 124*, 102158. https://doi.org/10.1016/j.artmed.2021.102158

Shekarchi, B., Panahi, A., Raeissadat, S., Maleki, N., Nayebabbas, S., & Farhadi, P. (2020). Comparison of Thessaly test with joint line tenderness and Mcmurray test in the diagnosis of meniscal tears. *Malaysian Orthopaedic Journal, 14*(2), 94–100. https://doi.org/10.5704/MOJ.2007.018

Slack, S. K., & Barclay, L. (2023). First-person disavowals of digital phenotyping and epistemic injustice in psychiatry. *Medicine, Health Care and Philosophy, 26*(4), 605–614. https://doi.org/10.1007/s11019-023-10174-8

Spencer, L. J. (2023). Hermeneutical injustice and unworlding in psychopathology. *Philosophical Psychology, 36*(7), 1300–1325. https://doi.org/10.1080/09515089.2023.2166821

Stone, A. A., & Shiffman, S. (1994). Ecological momentary assessment (Ema) in behavioral medicine. *Annals of Behavioral Medicine, 16*(3), 199–202. https://doi.org/10.1093/abm/16.3.199

Torous, J., Kiang, M. V., Lorme, J., & Onnela, J.-P. (2016). New tools for new research in psychiatry: A scalable and customizable platform to empower data driven smartphone research. *JMIR Mental Health, 3*(2), e5165. https://doi.org/10.2196/mental.5165

Williamson, S. (2023). Digital phenotyping in psychiatry. *BJPsych Advances, 29*(6), 428–429. https://doi.org/10.1192/bja.2023.26

Wolfers, T., Doan, N. T., Kaufmann, T., Alnæs, D., Moberget, T., Agartz, I., Buitelaar, J. K., Ueland, T., Melle, I., Franke, B., Andreassen, O. A., Beckmann, C. F., Westlye, L. T., & Marquand, A. F. (2018). Mapping the heterogeneous phenotype of schizophrenia and bipolar disorder using normative models. *JAMA Psychiatry, 75*(11), 1146–1155. https://doi.org/10.1001/jamapsychiatry.2018.2467

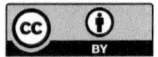

Index

© The Editor(s) (if applicable) and The Author(s) 2025
L. Bortolotti (ed.), *Epistemic Justice in Mental Healthcare*,
https://doi.org/10.1007/978-3-031-68881-2

159